Nursing Drug Dosages and their Calculations

Nursing Drug Dosages and their Calculations

GL Chattri MBBS MD MHA
Consultant Pediatrician and Neonatologist
Metro Multispeciality Hospital and
Seth Mannulal Jagannath Hospital
Jabalpur, Madhya Pradesh, India

Foreword
Mahesh Maheshwari

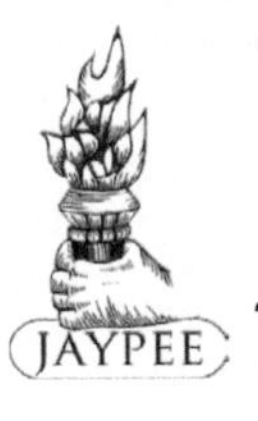

The Health Sciences Publisher
New Delhi | London | Panama

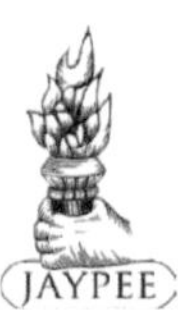

JAYPEE **Jaypee Brothers Medical Publishers (P) Ltd**

Headquarters

Jaypee Brothers Medical Publishers (P) Ltd
4838/24, Ansari Road, Daryaganj
New Delhi 110 002, India
Phone: +91-11-43574357
Fax: +91-11-43574314
Email: jaypee@jaypeebrothers.com

Overseas Offices

J.P. Medical Ltd
83 Victoria Street, London
SW1H 0HW (UK)
Phone: +44 20 3170 8910
Fax: +44 (0)20 3008 6180
Email: info@jpmedpub.com

Jaypee-Highlights Medical Publishers Inc
City of Knowledge, Bld. 235, 2nd Floor, Clayton
Panama City, Panama
Phone: +1 507-301-0496
Fax: +1 507-301-0499
Email: cservice@jphmedical.com

Jaypee Brothers Medical Publishers (P) Ltd
17/1-B Babar Road, Block-B, Shaymali
Mohammadpur, Dhaka-1207, Bangladesh
Mobile: +08801912003485
Email: jaypeedhaka@gmail.com

Jaypee Brothers Medical Publishers (P) Ltd
Bhotahity, Kathmandu, Nepal
Phone +977-9741283608
Email: kathmandu@jaypeebrothers.com

Website: www.jaypeebrothers.com
Website: www.jaypeedigital.com

Nursing Drug Dosages and their Calculations

First Edition: **2017**

ISBN: 978-93-86261-07-6

Printed at Repro India Limited

Dedicated

To my loving family;

Rashmi
my wonderful wife, my best friend,
for her support and encouragement,
I love coming home to you.

Dhruv and Shlok
my sons, who complete my life.

To the consummate pediatrician
Late (Prof) Dr VJ Rajpoot,
who taught me the art of pediatrics.

CONTRIBUTORS

Deepti Pandey MSc
(Medical Surgical Nursing)
Principal
Bhagyoday Tirth Nursing College
Sagar, Madhya Pradesh, India

Mahesh Maheshwari MBBS MD
(Pediatrics)
Associate Professor
People's Medical College
Bhopal, Madhya Pradesh, India

Malti Lodhi PhD (Pediatric Nursing)
Principal
Jabalpur Institute of Medical Science and Research
Jabalpur, Madhya Pradesh, India

Prerna Pandey MSc
(Pediatric Nursing)
Principal
SAIMS and College of Nursing
Indore, Madhya Pradesh, India

Sameer Agarwal MBBS DCH
(Pediatrics)
Senior Consultant
Sutika Grah Hospital
Jabalpur, Madhya Pradesh, India

Sapna Das MSc (Psychiatric Nursing)
Principal
Jabalpur Institute of
Nursing Science and Research
Jabalpur, Madhya Pradesh, India

Sini Shaji MSc (Psychiatric Nursing)
Professor
Mar Baselios College of Nursing
Bhopal, Madhya Pradesh, India

Swarnlata Peter MSc
(Medical Surgical Nursing)
Principal
Regional Institute of Nursing
Jabalpur, Madhya Pradesh, India

FOREWORD

I am privileged to write the foreword of Dr GL Chattri's *Nursing Drug Dosages and their Calculations*, which I believe, is a pioneering work in the field.

Nursing is one of the most vital aspects of the medical profession. Nursing education is concerned with the delivery of knowledge, attitude and practice to the future generation.

In 55 well-written chapters by the authors, I find that chapters were classified on the basis of group of drugs, further described in various headings including drug action, uses, available brand names, side effects. Nursing consideration is well-illustrated by explaining—what to assess, how to administer, advice and desired outcome of drug in an understandable language. There are separate chapters on weight and measures, calculation of drug dosages and pediatric drug dosages calculation.

Each and every chapter is peer-reviewed, evidence-based and state-of-the-art. The descriptions are reader-friendly, easy-to-follow and profusely supported by updated literature.

In order to further enhance the usefulness of the book, appendices are annexed towards the conclusion of the book to provide the access to a wide range of important information relevant to the drug dosages in the form of practically useful charts and tables and diagrams.

Hopefully, the book with most advance knowledge shall prove useful to the readers.

Dr Mahesh Maheshwari
Professor, Pediatrics
People's College of Medical Sciences and Research
Bhopal, Madhya Pradesh, India
People's University
Bhopal, Madhya Pradesh, India
drmaheshkiran@gmail.com

FOREWORD

PREFACE

I am pleased to have an opportunity to write this book *Nursing Drug Dosages and their Calculations*. It is essential that nursing students, nurses and other health care providers should know more than the names and doses of drugs they are administering. This book is designed to be a practical and convenient guide to dose calculation and administration of medication in adults and pediatric patients, along with basic information of each drug (action, uses, brands, side effects and nursing considerations). Since it is not possible to cover everything in a small book, a few groups and drugs may be missing.

Book is organized in two sections—Section 1 containing drug details based on therapeutic and pharmacological classification, Section 2 containing information on calculation of drug dosages under practically useful headings.

Dosages vary with the age, weight, surface area and disease, etc. Overdosing may lead to side effects and underdosing will lead to unsatisfactory response or development of resistance in cases of antibiotics.

Though all efforts have been made to avert any error in the text, drug doses and calculation of drug dosages; still any inadvertent error may creep in. In case of any doubt about any section, always check with another standard book. Due to everyday research it is advised to consult package insert before using drug.

This book will be very useful for the nursing students, practicing nurses and other health care providers. Nurses will be more confident in understanding drugs, calculating and administering medicines and will be able to provide care to their patients in a better way.

GL Chattri

ACKNOWLEDGMENTS

First of all, I would like to thank my parents whose blessings made my dream come true, and special thanks to my wife and kids, who spare me to spend, from their share of valuable time, in writing this book. My wife is always a source of encouragement for me.

I express my deep gratitude to Mr Sanjeev Pandey, for typing the manuscript, and his personal support.

I sincerely thank Shri Jitendar P Vij (Group Chairman), Mr Ankit Vij (Group President), Ms Chetna Malhotra Vohra (Associate Director-Content Strategy) and staff of Jaypee Brothers Medical Publishers, for publishing the book.

My special thanks to my friends Dr Sameer Agarwal and Dr Mahesh Maheswari for their professional help, guidance and support.

HOW TO USE THE BOOK

SECTION 1

Medication informations are provided in a below mentioned format and covered in short to make the book user-friendly. All components may not appear in each drug/section:

- **Therapeutic classification:** Drugs are classified by the disease state for which they are used, e.g. Analgesics
- **Pharmacological classification:** Drugs are further classified based on mechanism of action, e.g. Analgesics—non-narcotics
- **Generic name:** Indian adopted names of individual drug, e.g. Acetaminophen
- **Action:** Contains in short how the drug produces its effect
- **Uses:** Contains information about the common diseases or condition for which the drug is used
- **Dosage:** Includes recommended doses for adult and pediatric patients
- **Brands:** Contains information about strength and concentration of available forms and trade names
- **Side effects:** Since it is not possible to include all reported reactions, only common and serious ones are included
- **Nursing considerations:** Contains informations that nursing staff and patients and/or families of patient should know about drug usage and includes the following:
  - *Assessment:* Includes physical examination, laboratory investigation, history which should be elicited before and during therapy
  - *Administration:* Contains information about how and when to administer drug (route, diluents, rate, concentration, reconstitution, etc.)
  - *Advise:* Information that patient and/or families should know or to be taught by nurses to them about drug usage, reporting information, home care issues, follow-up requirements, additional nonpharmacological therapy that can be combined, etc.
  - *Desired outcome (DO):* Includes information to determine the effectiveness of drug therapy and patient response.

If more than one drug shares action, uses, side effects or nursing considerations, then instead of repetition with individual drugs, they are given together along with either pharmacological or therapeutic classification and therefore information applies to all drugs of a group if information is not given with individual drug.

SECTION 2

In this section, information about calculation of drug dosages is given under practically useful headings as follows:

- **Learning basic mathematics:** Basic mathematics knowledge required while calculating and understanding drugs order
- **Weights and measures:** Various weights and measures used, their symbols and conversion from one unit to another are explained
- **Calculating drug dosages:** Various methods used to calculate drug dosages are explained
- **Calculating pediatric drug dosages:** Calculating pediatric dose from the known adult dosage is explained
- **Calculating maintenance fluid requirement in children:** Methods based on body weight and body surface area are explained
- **IV drip rate calculation:** Calculating drip rate per hour or minutes from the ordered dose is explained
- **Administering medicines to children:** Contains practically useful tips helpful in administering medicines to pediatric patients
- **Solving problems:** A few problems are set-up for solving, based on the methods explained and learned.

CONTENTS

SECTION 1: NURSING DRUG DOSES

SECTION 2: CALCULATION OF DRUG DOSAGES

SYMBOLS AND ABBREVIATIONS

ACE	Angiotensin Converting Enzyme
Adm	Administration
AF	Atrial Fibrillation
AIDS	Acquired Immunodeficiency Syndrome
AOM	Acute Otitis Media
APD	Action Potential Duration
APTT	Activated Partial Thromboplastin Time
ARDS	Adult Respiratory Distress Syndrome
ARF	Acute Renal Failure
Assess	Assessment
AV	Atrioventricular
AZT	Azathioprine
BD	Twice Daily
BM	Bone Marrow
BP	Blood Pressure
BPD	Bronchopulmonary Dysplasia
BPH	Benign Prostatic Hypertrophy
BT	Bleeding Time
CAP	Community Acquired Pneumonia
CBC	Complete Blood Count
CD4	Helper T4 Lymphocyte Cells
CHD	Congenital Heart Disease
CHF	Congestive Heart Failure
C/I	Contraindications
CK	Creatinine Kinase
CMV	Cytomegalovirus
CNS	Central Nervous System
CO	Cardiac Output
COPD	Chronic Obstructive Pulmonary Disease
CP	Cerebral Palsy
CPK	Creatinine Phosphokinase
CPR	Cardiopulmonary Resuscitation
CPS	Complex Partial Seizures
CR	Cardiorespiratory
CRF	Chronic Renal Failure
C/S	Culture and Sensitivity

CSF	Cerebrospinal Fluid
CTZ	Chemoreceptor Trigger Zone
CV	Cardiovascular
CxR	Chest X-Ray
DM	Diabetes Mellitus
DNS	Dextrose Normal Saline
DO	Desired Outcome
DUB	Dysfunctional Uterine Bleeding
D_5W	Dextrose 5% Water
$D_{10}W$	Dextrose 10% Water
EC	Enteric Coated
ECG	Electrocardiogram
EEG	Electroencephalogram
e.g.	For Example
EPS	Extrapyramidal Symptoms
ERP	Effective Refractory Period
ET	Endotracheal
FA	Folic Acid
FDP	Fibrinogen Degradation Products
FS	Focal Seizures
GA	General Anesthesia
GABA	Gamma Aminobutyric Acid
GERD	Gastroesophageal Reflux Disease
GI	Gastrointestinal
GIT	Gastrointestinal Tract
gm	Gram
G6PD	Glucose 6 Phosphate Dehydrogenase
GTCS	Generalized Tonic Clonic Seizures
GU	Genitourinary
GUTI	Genitourinary Tract Infection
HA	Headache
Hb	Hemoglobin
HDL	High Density Lipoproteins
HDN	Hemorrhagic Disease of Newborn
HIV	Human Immunodeficiency Virus
H/O	History of
HR	Heart Rate
hr	Hour
HS	At Bedtime
HSV	Herpes Simplex Virus

IBS	Irritable Bowel Syndrome
ICH	Intracranial Hemorrhage
ICP	Intracranial Pressure
IM	Intramuscular
I/O	Input and Output
IOP	Intraocular Pressure
ITP	Idiopathic Thrombocytopenic Purpura
IU	International Unit
IV	Intravenous
IVP	Intravenous Push
JVP	Jugular Venous Pressure
Kg	Kilogram
L	Liter
LFT	Liver Function Test
LRTI	Lower Respiratory Tract Infection
m^2	Square Meter
MAO	Monoamine Oxidase
max	Maximum
mcg/µg	Microgram
MDI	Metered Dose Inhaler
mEq	Milli Equivalent
mg	Milligram
MI	Myocardial Infarction
min	Minute
ml	Milliliter
mm^3	Cubic Millimeter
MS	Multiple Sclerosis
mth	Month
NB	Newborn
NC	Nursing Considerations
NEC	Necrotising Enterocolitis
NG	Nasogastric
NMS	Neuroleptic Malignant Syndrome
NS	Normal Saline
NSAID	Nonsteroidal Anti-Inflammatory Drug
N/V	Nausea and Vomiting
OA	Osteoarthritis
OCD	Obsessive Compulsive Disorder
OD	Once Daily
OM	Otitis Media

Oz	Ounce
PDA	Patent Ductus Arteriosus
PFT	Pulmonary Function Test
PID	Pelvic Inflammatory Disease
PO	Per Oral/By Mouth
PP	Peripheral Pulses
PS	Partial Seizures
PSE	Portosystemic Encephalopathy
PSVT	Paroxysmal Supraventricular Tachycardia
PTH	Parathyroid Hormone
PVC	Premature Ventricular Contractions
q	Every
QID	Every Four Hourly
RC	Rectal
RFT	Renal Function Test
RL	Ringer Lactate
R/O	Rule Out
ROP	Retinopathy of Prematurity
RR	Respiratory Rate
RSV	Respiratory Syncytial Virus
RTI	Respiratory Tract Infection
SA	Sinoatrial
SC	Subcutaneous
S/E	Side Effects
SJS	Stevens Johnson Syndrome
SL	Sublingual
SLE	Systemic Lupus Erythematosus
SPS	Simple Partial Seizures
S/S	Signs and Symptoms
SSRIs	Selective Serotonin Reuptake Inhibitors
SSTI	Skin and Soft Tissue Infection
STD	Sexually Transmitted Disease
SVT	Supraventricular Tachycardia
SVTA	Supraventricular Tachyarrhythmia
SWI	Sterile Water for Injection
TB	Tuberculosis
TDS	Thrice Daily
TG	Triglycerides
TIA	Transient Ischemic Attack
U/O	Urine Output

URTI	Upper Respiratory Tract Infection
UTI	Urinary Tract Infection
VF	Ventricular Fibrillation
wk	Week
wt	Weight
>	Greater than
≥	Greater than or Equal to
<	Lesser than
≤	Lesser than or Equal to
–ve	Negative
+ve	Positive
%	Percent
/	Per
+	With, Positive (as applicable)
±	With or Without

Section 1

Nursing Drug Doses

A dose is the amount of drug administered in various forms at one time. The minimum dose is the smallest quantity of the drug that will produce the desired effect. The maximum dose is the largest quantity of the drug that can be given at one time for desired effect without producing any harm to the body.

Chapter 1

Analgesics

Includes: (A) Non-narcotics and (B) Narcotics

(A) ANALGESICS—NON-NARCOTICS

1. Acetaminophen/Paracetamol
2. Aspirin/Acetylsalicylic acid
3. Benzocaine
4. Bupivacaine
5. Capsaicin
6. Diclofenac
7. Flurbiprofen
8. Ibuprofen
9. Indomethacin
10. Ketoprofen
11. Ketorolac
12. Lidocaine
13. Mefenamic acid
14. Meloxicam
15. Naproxen
16. Phenazopyridine
17. Piroxicam

Action: Majority of non-narcotic analgesics acts by inhibiting prostaglandin synthesis peripherally for analgesic effect and centrally for antipyretic effect. Aspirin also decreases platelet aggregation.

Uses: To control mild to moderate pain and/or fever. Aspirin is also useful for inflammatory conditions; RA and OA, TIA and MI. Phenazopyridine as urinary tract analgesic and capsaicin as topical analgesic.

Side Effects: Serious side effects include; nephrotoxicity, hepatitis, blood dyscrasias and common being; nausea, abdominal pain, dizziness, drowsiness.

General Nursing Considerations

- **Assess:** RFT, LFT, hematocrit, BT, PT especially in patient on chronic use; input and output, decreased output may indicate renal failure. Blurred vision, ringing in ears, change in urine pattern, increased weight, edema for drug toxicity. Look for history of allergies, asthma, as these patients are at increased risk of hypersensitivity reactions. Anti-inflammatory effect require higher dosage as compared to that required for analgesia and pain relief. NSAIDs may inhibit the cardioprotective effects of aspirin.
- **Administration:** With food or an antacid or after meals to prevent gastric irritation. Do not crush, break or allow chewing of sustained release preparations. Topical preparations should be applied to intact skin with maximum pain. Do not allow antacids within 1–2 hours of enteric coated tablets.

- **Advise:** Taking plenty of water and remaining in sitting position for 15–30 minutes after intake. To wear protective clothing and sunscreen to avoid photosensitivity reactions, avoid using contact lenses while using ophthalmic solutions. Periodic eye and ear check-up for patients on chronic therapy. Regularly administered doses are more effective than SOS doses. To avoid concomitant use of alcohol as it increases risk of GI hemorrhage, and to report in case of bleeding, eye symptoms, tinnitus, purpura, decreased urine output.
- Geriatric patients are at increased risk of side effects, so use lowest effective doses. Patient who do not respond to one may respond to another NSAIDs. Explaining the therapeutic value of medication before administration enhances the analgesic effect. Analgesia is better controlled if drug given before pain becomes severe. These agents may need to be withheld before surgery.

1. Acetaminophen/Paracetamol

Uses: Pain, fever.

Dosage:

- Adults (PO, RC): 325–650 mg every 4–6 hours (Max: 4 g/day)
- Infants and children (PO, RC): 10–20 mg/kg/dose every 4–6 hours as needed
- Neonates (PO, RC): 10–15 mg/kg/dose every 6–8 hours
- Adults and children (IM): 5 mg/kg/dose.

Brands: 500, 650 mg Tabs; 125, 250 mg/5 ml Syp; Medomol, Pacimol, T-98. 150 mg/mL Inj; Febrinil, Paracip. 80, 170, 250 mg suppository; Anamol, Paracetanal.

Side Effects: Hepatotoxicity, hepatic failure.

Nursing Considerations: In diabetic patients it may result in false rise in urine glucose and fall in serum glucose levels. Rate of absorption is decreased if given with food rich in carbohydrates. To be used with caution in G6PD deficiency cases.

2. Aspirin/Acetylsalicylic Acid

Uses: Pain, fever, arthritis, rheumatic fever, TIA, MI.

Dosage: PO

- Pain, fever; Adults: 325–1000 mg every 4–6 hours. Children >2 years: 10–15 mg/kg every 4–6 hours (Max: 4 g/day)
- Arthritis; Adults: 2.4 g/day initially in divided doses, maintenance dose is 3.6–5.4 g/day. Children: 60–90 mg/kg/day in divided doses
- TIA, MI; Adults: 50–325 mg once daily (given indefinitely).

Brands: 75, 150 mg Tabs; Ecosprin, Delisprin, Zosprin.

Side Effects: GI bleeding, hepatitis, thrombocytopenia, tinnitus, convulsions.

Nursing Considerations: Monitor patients for tinnitus, headache, hyperventilation, diarrhea, sweating, black tarry stool, bleeding gums; if any of these occurs withhold the drug. If tablet smells like vinegar, discard it. Chronic use results in folic acid, iron and vitamin C deficiency; hypernatremia.

3. Benzocaine

Action: Blocks nerve conduction by decreasing membrane permeability to sodium ions.

Uses: Toothache, sore throat pain, hemorrhoids, rectal fissures, lubricant and analgesic for passage of catheter and endoscopic tubes.

Dosage: Use as required.

Brands: 7.5% gel; T-JEL.

Nursing Considerations: Do not administer orally for >2 days and do not use in children <2 years. Do not eat for 1 hour after oral use.

4. Bupivacaine

Action: Refer benzocaine.

Uses: Local, regional, spinal anesthesia or analgesia.

Dosage:

- Epidural: Adults and children ≥ 12 years: 10–20 ml of 0.25–0.75% solution

  Children <12 years: 1.25 mg/kg/dose
- Peripheral nerve block: 5 ml dose of 0.25 or 0.5% solution.

Brands: 0.25, 0.5% Inj; Bupivan, Sensorcaine. 1.0% Inj. Marcain.

Side Effects: Anxiety, arrhythmias, seizures, hypotension, urinary retention, bradycardia.

Nursing Considerations: Monitor BP, HR, RR continuously. Assess for systemic toxicity (circumoral tingling, ringing in ears, numbness, blurred vision, twitching). Solution containing preservative should not be used for epidural or caudal block.

5. Capsaicin

Action: Induces release of substance -P responsible for carrying impulses from periphery to CNS. After repeated application, neurons gets depleted of this substance.

Uses: Topically for arthritis, postherpetic neuralgia, diabetic neuropathy, postoperative pain.

Dosage: Adults and children >2 years: Apply to affected area 3–4 times/day.

Brands: 0.075% cream; Capsain.

Side Effects: Cough, transient burning.

Nursing Considerations: Rub after application so that no cream is left over. Transient burning occurs on initial application, which will decrease after few days of continuous use. In herpes zoster cases apply only after lesions are healed completely.

6. Diclofenac

Uses: Pain, arthritis; ophthalmic: postoperative inflammation; topical: actinic keratosis in adults.

Dosage:

- Adults (PO): 50–75 mg twice daily or thrice daily
- Children (PO): 2–3 mg/kg/day divided every 4 hours
- Ophthalmic: 1 drop of 0.1% solution 4 times/day
- Topical: Apply twice daily

Brands:

- Diclofenac Sodium: 50, 100 mg Tabs; 25 mg/mL Inj; Diclomax. Voveran.
- Diclofenac Potassium: 50 mg Tab; Knac, Volini. 0.1% eyedrops; Dicol, Fegan. 1.0% gel; Artifen-D, Deeclo.

Side Effects: GI bleeding, hepatitis, dyspepsia, tinnitus, hematuria, renal failure, bronchospasm.

Nursing Considerations: For rapid effect first dose can be taken empty stomach.

7. Flurbiprofen

Uses: Arthritis; Ophthalmic: postoperative inflammation.

Dosage:

- Adults (PO): 100–300 mg/day divided every 6–8 hours
- Ocular: 1 drop of 0.03% solution every 30 minutes starting 2 hours prior to surgery (total 4 drops) to each affected eyes

Brands: 100 mg Tab; Flurofen, Froben. 0.03% drops; FBN, Flur.

Side Effects: Refer Diclofenac.

8. Ibuprofen

Uses: Pain, fever, arthritis, dysmenorrhea.

Dosage: PO

- Pain and fever: Adults: 200–400 mg/dose every 4–6 hours.
  Children: 4–10 mg/kg/day divided every 6 hours.
- Arthritis: Adults: 400–800 mg/dose every 6–8 hours.
  Children: 30–50 mg/kg/day divided every 6 hours.

Brands: 200, 400, 600 mg Tabs; Brufen, Emflan, Ibugesic. 100 mg/5 ml susp; Bren, Ibugesic.

Side Effects: Refer Diclofenac

Nursing Considerations: Assess: Signs and symptoms of GI bleeding (black tarry stools, hypotension), renal dysfunction (increased urea and creatinine, decreased urine output), hepatic dysfunction (increased liver enzymes and bilirubin). Avoid usage in dehydrated patients as it may increase risk of renal dysfunction.

9. Indomethacin

Uses: Arthritis, PDA closure in neonates.

Dosage:

- Adults (PO): 25–50 mg 2–4 times/day
- Children (PO): 1–2 mg/kg/day divided every 6–12 hours
- Neonates; PDA closure: IV
  <2 days: 0.2 mg/kg, then 0.1 mg/kg after 12 and 24 hours
  2–7 days: 0.2 mg/kg, then 0.2 mg/kg after 12 and 24 hours
  >7 days: 0.2 mg/kg, then 0.25 mg/kg after 12 and 24 hours

Brands: 75 mg Tabs; Indoflam TR, Microcid. 25, 50 mg cap; Artisid, Indocap. 75 mg Inj; Donica.

Side Effects: GI bleeding, dizziness, hepatitis, constipation, skin allergy, edema, anaphylaxis.

Nursing Considerations: While using for PDA monitor BP, HR, ECG, respiratory status, input and output. For chronic therapy use lowest effective dose. For IV use dilute in normal saline or sterile water in a concentration of 0.5–1 mg/mL and use immediately after reconstitution, infuse over half an hour. Do not give via umbilical catheter.

10. Ketoprofen

Uses: Pain, fever, arthritis, dysmenorrhea.

Dosage: Adults (PO):

- Arthritis: 50–300 mg/day divided every 6–8 hours
- Analgesic: 25–50 mg every 6–8 hours

Brands: 50, 100 Tabs; Redufen. 50 mg cap; Ostofen.

Side Effects: Refer Indomethacin

Nursing Considerations: Urine albumin, bilirubin levels are altered.

11. Ketorolac

Uses: Short-term management of pain (<5 days); Ophthalmic: ocular pain associated with allergies or surgery.

Dosage:

- Adults (PO): 10 mg every 6–8 hours (Max: 40 mg/day)
- (IM, IV): 15–30 mg every 6 hours
- Ocular (Adults, Children >3 years): 1 drop of 0.4–0.5% solution

Brands: 10 mg Tab; Cadolac, Ketanov, Torolac. 0.5% eyedrops; Acular, Cadolac, Ketanov.

Side Effects: GI bleeding, drowsiness, allergy.

Nursing Considerations: Use PO only as continuation of IV/IM therapy. For IV dilute as 15–30 mg/mL in NS, DNS, D_5%, RL and infuse over 30 seconds. Color change indicate degradation. Apply pressure over lacrimal sac for 20 minutes after application to avoid systemic absorption. Use lower doses in elderly, renal patients <50 kg weight.

12. Lidocaine

Action: Blocks nerve conduction by decreasing membrane permeability to sodium ions.

Uses: Topical/local anesthetic, relief of pain in postherpetic neuralgia.

Dosage: Adults and Children:
- Infilteration: Apply to affected areas as needed (Max: 4.5 mg/kg/dose)
- Topical: Apply as needed (Max: 3 mg/kg/dose)
- Patch: 1–3 patch/day
- Mucosal: 10–15 ml of viscous solution every 3 hours for oral or pharyngeal pain. Male urethra, 3–5 ml and female urethra 5–10 ml of jelly.

Brands: 1, 2% Inj, 2,5% jelly; 5% oint; Xylocaine, Gesicain.

Side Effects: Anaphylaxis, cardiac arrest, seizures, confusion, drowsiness, hypotension.

Nursing Considerations: Epinephrine may be combined with Lidocaine to minimize systemic absorption and prolong local effect. Oral spray and solution may impair swallowing, so ensure that gag reflex is intact before allowing patient to take orally. For dermal procedure apply cream 2 hours prior. For infiltration or topical use don't repeat within 2 hours.

13. Mefenamic Acid

Uses: Pain, fever, arthritis, dysmenorrhea.

Dosage: PO: Should not be given for >1 week
- Adults: 250–500 mg thrice daily
- Children: Fever; 3 mg/kg/dose twice daily. Arthritis; 10–25 mg/kg/day every 6 hours

Brands: 250, 500 mg Tabs; Meftal, Ponstan. 50 mg/5 mL susp; Ponstan.

14. Meloxicam

Uses: Arthritis.

Dosage: PO
- Adults: 7.5–15 mg once daily
- Children > 2 years < 12 kg: 0.125 mg/kg once daily (Max: 7.5 mg/day).

Brands: 7.5, 15 mg Tab; Melfan, Movac.

15. Naproxen

Uses: Fever, pain, arthritis, dysmenorrhea.

Dosage: PO
- Adults: 250–500 mg twice daily
- Children > 2 years: 5–7 mg/kg/dose every 8–12 hours.

Brands: 250 mg Tab; Nalyxan, Napryn.

16. Phenazopyridine

Uses: Urinary frequency, burning, itching in association with UTI or following urologic procedure.

Dosage: PO

- Adults: 100–200 mg/day in 3 divided doses
- Children: 12 mg/kg/day in 3 divided doses.

Brands: 200 mg Tab; Pyridactil, Pyridium.

Side Effects: Orange red urine, headache, rash, dizziness, GI disturbances, methemoglobinemia.

Nursing Considerations: Concurrent antibiotics must be taken and should be given only for 2 days. Administer after meals and tablet should be swallowed whole. It may cause orange red discoloration of urine that may stain clothing and bedding. Soft contact lenses may be stained. Interferes with urinary tests based on color, e.g. bilirubin, protein, glucose, ketones. Treatment should be discontinued if skin or sclera becomes yellow in color.

17. Piroxicam

Uses: Pain, arthritis.

Dosage: PO

- Adults: 10–20 mg/day twice daily
- Children: 0.2–0.3 mg/kg/day once daily (Max: 15 mg/day).

Brands: 10, 20 mg Tabs; Brexic, Paricam. 10, 20 mg cap; Toldin, Pirox.

(B) ANALGESICS—NARCOTICS

1. Buprenorphine
2. Butorphanol
3. Codeine
4. Dextropropoxyphene
5. Fentanyl
6. Meperidine/Pethidine
7. Morphine
8. Pentazocine
9. Tramadol

Action: They act by binding to opiate receptors in the CNS thereby decreasing pain impulse transmission.

Uses: Moderate to severe pain, some agents also used as adjunct to anesthesia.

Side Effects: Common side effects are—nausea, vomiting, anorexia, hypotension, constipation, cramps, headache, dizziness, sedation. Serious side effects include—respiratory depression, respiratory arrest, circulatory depression, raised intracranial pressure.

General Nursing Considerations

- **Assess:** BP, PR, respiration before and during administration; input and output, urinary retention, dysuria. When increasing doses, specially monitor respiratory status and level of consciousness
- **Administration:** To increase the analgesic effect explain patient about the therapeutic benefits of drug before administration. Analgesic effect is enhanced if given before pain becomes severe. Give with antiemetics if nausea and vomiting occurs. Hypoventilation can be prevented by physical stimulations and dose needs to be decreased. Always withdraw drug slowly to avoid withdrawal symptoms. Co-administration with NSAIDs

may increase analgesic effects and permit lower narcotic doses. Narcotics depress cough reflex. Turn every 2 hourly; cough and deep breathe to prevent atelectasis. If RR is <12/min. or the systolic blood pressure is <90 mm Hg, a narcotic should not be used unless there is ventilatory support

- **Advise:** Avoid activities requiring alertness while on narcotic therapy. To prevent orthostatic hypotension, change position slowly. Constipation can be prevented by increased intake of bulk foods, fluids or by use of laxatives or stool softeners. To decrease dry mouth symptoms; maintain good oral hygiene, frequent oral rinses. Advocate chest physiotherapy and breathing exercises to prevent atelectasis. May cause physical and psychological dependence, drowsiness. Initial drowsiness will diminish with continued use
- **Desired outcome:** Control of pain.

1. Buprenorphine

Uses: Moderate to severe pain, treatment of opioid dependence.

Dosage:

- Adults (IM, IV): 0.3 mg every 4–6 hours as needed, may be repeated after 30 minutes
- (SL):12–16 mg/day as a single dose.

Brands: 0.2 mg Tab; Tidigesic. 0.3 mg/ml Inj; Buprigesic, Norphin.

Side Effects: Hallucinations, dysphoria, sweating.

Nursing Considerations: Do not chew or swallow SL tab. Compatible with NS/D_5W/RL, may be given IV undiluted but should be given very slowly as rapid IV push may cause respiratory depression, cardiac arrest, hypotension.

2. Butorphenol

Uses: Pain, adjunct to anesthesia.

Dosage:

- Adults: (IM): 2 mg every 3–4 hours as needed
- (IV): 1 mg every 3–4 hours as needed.

Brands: 1, 2 mg/mL Inj; Butrum, Butadol.

Side Effects: Refer Buprenorphine.

Nursing Considerations: IV can be given undiluted over 3–5 minutes at a rate of 1 mg/min as rapid infusion may cause respiratory depression, hypotension, cardiac arrest.

3. Codeine

Uses: Pain, non-productive cough.

Dosage:

- Pain: Adults (PO): 15–30 mg/dose every 4–6 hours.
  Children (PO): 0.5–1 mg/kg/dose every 4–6 hours (Max: 60 mg/dose).

- Antitussive: Adults (PO): 10–20 mg every 4–6 hours.
  Children (PO) >2 year: 1–1.5 mg/kg/dose divided every 4–6 hours.

Brands: Available in combination. Codeine phosphate 10 mg + CPM 4 mg/5 ml Syp; Ascoril-C, Zenodyl.

4. Dextropropoxyphene

Uses: Mild to moderate pain.

Dosage: PO

- Adults: 65 mg every 4 hours (Max: 390 mg/day)
- Children: 2–3 mg/kg/day divided every 6 hours.

Brands: Available in combinations.

- Dextropropoxyphene + Paracetamol: 65 + 650 mg Tab; Dexovon, Lupivon.
- Dextropropoxyphene + Ibuprofen: 65 + 400 mg Cap; Lobain, Parvon forte.

5. Fentanyl

Uses: Pain, sedation, preoperative medication, adjunct to anesthesia, chronic pain (transdermal patch).

Dosage:

- Adults and Children > 12 years:
  Preoperative sedation (IV, IM): 50–100 μg/dose
  Adjunct to general anesthesia (IV, IM): 2–50 μg/kg
  Analgesia (IV): 0.5–1 μg/kg/dose, may be repeated after 1/2–1 hours
  Transdermal patch: Initial 25 μg/hours system, dose may be increased after 3 days (patch usually lasts for 48–72 hour).

Side Effects: Apnea, laryngospasm, sweating.

Brands: 50 μg/ml Inj; Fendrop, Fent. 25, 50, 100 μg/hours patch; Duragesic.

Nursing Considerations:

- For IV, 50 μg/ml can be given slowly over 5–10 minutes diluted is NS or D_5%. Always give slowly as rapid infusion may result in skeletal muscle and chest wall rigidity, impaired ventilation, respiratory distress, apnea, bronchospasm
- Patch: Always apply to non hairy, clean, dry, non irritated and non irradiated site such as chest, back, flank, upper arm. Apply immediately after opening pack. Do not apply new patch to same site. Do not use soap, alcohol to remove patch; use plain water only. Fever, heating pads, hot tubs, heated water beds increase the release of drug from the patch.

6. Meperidine/Pethidine

Uses: Pain, preoperative sedation, adjunct to anesthesia.

Dosage: PO, IM, IV, SC.

- Adults: 50–150 mg every 3–4 hours as needed
- Children: 1–1.5 mg/kg/dose every 3–4 hours as needed (Max: 100 mg/dose).

Brands: 50 mg/ml Inj; Pethidine.

Nursing Considerations: IV can be given diluted in NS/D5W/RL in a concentration of 1 mg/ml, to be infused over 15–30 minutes. Rapid IV infusion may cause respiratory depression, hypotension, cardiac arrest.

7. Morphine

Uses: Severe pain, pulmonary edema, pain associated with MI.

Dosage:
- Adults (PO): 10–30 mg every 4 hours
- Children (PO): 0.2–0.5 mg/kg/dose every 4–6 hours.

Brands: 10 mg Tabs CR, 30 mg Tab; Duramor, Morcontin.

8. Pentazocine

Uses: Moderate to severe pain, sedative prior to surgery, supplement to surgical anesthesia.

Dosage:
- Adults (PO): 50 mg every 3–4 hours (Max: 600 mg/day)
  (IV, IM): 30–60 mg every 3–4 hours (Max: 360 mg/day)
- Children > 2 years (IV, IM): 0.5 mg/kg as a single dose.

Brands: 25 mg Tab; Fortwin. 30 mg/ml Inj; Fortwin, Susevin.

Side Effects: Hallucinations, dysphoria, sweating.

Nursing Considerations: IV can be given diluted in SWI in a concentration of 5 mg/ml, to be given at a rate of 5 mg/min.

9. Tramadol

Uses: Short-term control of moderate to severe pain.

Dosage:
- Adults (PO): 50–100 mg every 4–6 (Max: 300 mg/day)
  (IV, IM, SC): 25–50 mg as needed every 6–8 hours
- Children (PO): 1 mg/kg as needed every 6–8 hours.

Brands: 50, 100 mg Tabs; Inodol, Ubitol. 100 mg SR Tabs; Contromol, Dolotram. 50 mg Cap and 100 mg SR Caps: Adamon, Domadol. 50 mg/ml Inj; Contramal, Domadol.

Side Effects: Seizures, headache, drowsiness, somnolence, nausea, constipation, dry mouth, physical dependence.

Chapter 2 Anti-Alzheimer's Agents

Includes: 1. Donepezil
2. Galantamine
3. Memantine
4. Rivastigmine

Action: Increases the amount of acetylcholine in the CNS by inhibiting cholinesterase.

Use: Alzheimer's dementia.

Side Effects: Headache, dizziness, diarrhea, nausea, weight gain or loss.

General Nursing Considerations

- **Assess:** Monitor hypotension, hypertension, nausea and vomiting, anorexia, weight loss. Assess for memory, language, attention, depression, ability to perform simple tasks, urinary frequency, incontinence
- **Administration:** Give with antiemetic and adequate fluid to decrease nausea and vomiting. PO ± food. As most side effects occurs during increasing doses, increase gradually over 4 weeks
- **Advise:** To report any side effect. Inform patients and caregivers that improvement in cognitive functions may take weeks to month and the disease process is not reversible
- **Desired outcome:** Improvement in memory, language, attention.

1. Donepezil

Dosage: PO: Adults: 5 mg once daily, may be increased after 4–6 weeks to 10 mg once daily

Brands: 5, 10 mg Tabs; Alzil, Donaz, Donep.

2. Galantamine

Dosage: PO: Adults: 8–16 mg/day divided every 12 hours; start with lower doses and then increase gradually after 4 weeks.

Brands: 4, 8, 12 mg Tabs; Galamer.

3. Memantine

Dosage: PO: Adults: Initially 5 mg once daily, can be increased weekly to maximum of 20 mg once daily

Brands: 5, 10 mg Tabs; Admenta, Demezil.

4. Rivastigmine

Dosage: PO: Adults: Initial dose of 1.5 mg twice daily, can be increased after 2 weeks to 3 mg twice daily.

Brands: 1.5, 3, 4.5, 6 mg Tabs; Exelon, Rivamer.

Chapter

3 Antianginals

Includes: (A) Beta-blockers
(B) Calcium channel blockers
(C) Nitrates

(A) ANTIANGINALS—BETA-BLOCKERS

Includes: 1. Atenolol 2. Labetalol 3. Metoprolol 4. Propranolol

Action: Decreases myocardial oxygen consumption by decreasing heart rate.

Side Effects: Common side effects are; fatigue, headache, dizziness, nausea, drowsiness, diarrhea, postural hypotension, erectile dysfunction, bronchospasm. Serious side effects include; bradycardia, CHF, pulmonary edema, arrhythmias.

General Nursing Considerations

- **Assess:** BP, HR, ECG, I/O, daily weight, edema, chest pain. History of asthma, DM, impaired renal function; signs and symptoms of hypoglycemia, CHF
- **Administration:** Take pulse prior to giving drug, if heart rate <50/min, notify this to the doctor. They can be given with or without meals. Sudden withdrawal may precipitate or worsen angina, rebound HT, MI
- **Advise:** To take drug same time per day. Do not stop abruptly. Avoid activities requiring alertness. Change position slowly to minimize orthostatic hypotension. Sensitivity to cold may be increased. Inform if there is difficulty in breathing, wheezing, cold hands and feets, dizziness or confusion. Diabetic patient should monitor blood sugar daily. Avoid excessive intake of alcohol, coffee, tea or cola
- **Desired Outcome:** Decrease in BP and frequency of angina, prevention of MI, increase in activity tolerance.

1. Atenolol

Uses: Hypertension, angina pectoris, prevention of MI.

Dosage:

- Adults: PO: Antianginal; 50–100 mg once daily. Antihypertensive; 25–100 mg once daily for 6–9 days

- Children: PO: Initial 0.8–1 mg/kg/dose, can be titrated upto maximum of 100 mg/day.

Brands: 25, 50, 100 mg Tabs; Atecard, Aten, Betacard.

2. Labetalol

Uses: HT.

Dosage:

- Adults: PO: Initial 100 mg twice daily may be increased every 2–3 days by 100 mg as needed. IV: Initial 20 mg, 10 minutes later 20–40 mg may be given if required
- Children: PO: 4 mg/kg/day divided every 12 hours. IV: 0.2–1 mg/kg/day.

Brands: 10 mg Tabs; 5 mg/ml Inj; Lobet.

Nursing Consideration: IV can be given at the rate of 2 mg/min.

3. Metoprolol

Uses: HT, angina pectoris, prevention of MI.

Dosage:

- Adults (PO): Antihypertensive/Antianginal; 25–100 mg/day divided every 12 hours. MI; 25–50 mg every 6 hours for 48 hours, then 100 mg twice daily for 3 months
- Adults: (IV) MI; 5 mg every 2 minutes for 3 doses followed by oral doses.

Brands: 25, 50, 100 mg Tabs; 1 mg/ml Inj; Betaloc, Metolar.

Nursing Considerations: Give IV slowly over 2–5 minutes.

4. Propranolol

Uses: HT, angina pectoris, arrhythmias, prevention of MI.

Dosage:

- Adults: PO: Antianginal; 80–320 mg/day divided every 6 hours. Antihypertensive; 40 mg twice daily. Antiarrhythmic; 10–30 mg, 3–4 times/day. Prevention of MI; 180–240 mg/day in divided doses
- Adults: IV: Antiarrhythmic; Initial 1–3 mg, may be repeated after 2 minutes and 4 hours if needed
- Children: PO: Antihypertensive/Antiarrhythmic; 0.5–1 mg/kg/day divided every 6 hours
- Children: IV: 10–100 μg/kg (0.01–0.1 mg/kg) by slow IV.

Brands: 10, 40 mg Tabs; Ciplar, Corbeta. 1 mg/ml Inj; Properol.

Nursing Consideration: IV can be given at the rate of 0.5–1 mg/min.

(B) ANTIANGINALS—CALCIUM CHANNEL BLOCKERS

Include: 1. Diltiazem 2. Felodipine
3. Nifedipine 4. Verapamil

Action: Acts by dilating coronary arteries, some agents also slow down heart rate and suppresses ventricular tachyarrhythmias.

Uses: HT, angina pectoris, vasospastic angina. Diltiazem and verapamil in addition also used for supraventricular tachyarrhythmias.

Side Effects: Common side effects are: Headache, flushing, peripheral edema. Serious side effects include; CHF, arrhythmias, SJS.

General Nursing Considerations

- **Assess:** BP, HR, ECG, I/O, daily weight, serum potassium, chest pain. Signs and symptoms of CHF
- **Administration:** PO can be given with or without meals. As these drugs cause peripheral vasodilation, any excessive hypotensive response and increased heart rate may precipitate angina.
- **Advise:** Do not stop drug abruptly. Restrict exercise and avoid activities requiring alertness. Change position slowly to minimize orthostatic hypotension. Report dyspnea, swelling of extremities, headache, dizziness, hypotension. Combine other methods of lowering BP—low sodium diet, decrease weight, stop smoking and alcohol. Avoid long periods of standing, excessive heat, hot showers, may exacerbate drop in BP
- **Desired Outcome:** Decrease in BP, chest pain, need for nitrate therapy; increase in activity tolerance; suppression of arrhythmias.

1. Diltiazem

Dosage:
- Adults: PO: 30–120 mg 3–4 times/day
- Children: PO: 1.5–2 mg/kg/day divided every 8 hours

Brands: 30, 60, 90 mg Tabs; Dilcal, Dilzem.

2. Felodipine

Dosage: Adults: PO: 5 mg/day may be increased every 2 weeks to maximum of 10 mg/day

Brands: 2.5, 5, 10 mg Tabs; Felogard, Plendil.

3. Nifedipine

Dosage:
- Adults: PO: 10–30 mg 3 times/day
- Ped: PO: 0.25–0.5 mg/kg/dose (Max: 10 mg/day).

Brands: 5, 10 mg Tabs; Nifedine. 10, 20 mg Cap; Calcigard, Depin.

4. Verapamil

Dosage:
- Adults: PO: 80–120 mg, 3 times/day. IV: 5–10 mg may be repeated after 15–30 minutes.
- Children: > 16 years: PO: 4–8 mg/kg/day divided every 6–8 hours
  1–16 years: IV: 0.1–0.3 mg/kg/dose may be repeated after 30 minutes

Brands: 40, 80 mg Tabs; 2.5 mg/ml Inj; Calaptin.

(C) ANTIANGINALS—NITRATES

Include: 1. Isosorbide dinitrate 2. Isosorbide mononitrate
3. Nitroglycerine

Action: Causes coronary arteries dilatation and systemic vasodilatation.

Uses: Treatment and prevention of angina.

Side Effects: Headache, dizziness, nausea, dry mouth, tachycardia, hypotension, blurred vision.

General Nursing Considerations

- **Assess:** BP, HR, ECG, I/O, chest pain, any precipitating factors (stress, activity). History of anemia, administer with extreme caution
- **Administration:** SL tablets should be held under tongue. Drinking and eating should be avoided until its dissolves. Tolerance may develop on chronic use, manifested by absence of response to usual dose (discontinue temporarily and reinstitute later on). PO doses are taken empty stomach with water
- **Advise:** Do not stop abruptly. Change position slowly. Avoid activities requiring alertness. Take last dose before 7 pm to prevent development of tolerance. Report dry mouth and blurred vision. Avoid changing brands. Carry SL tablets in a glass bottle, tightly capped. If pain is not relieved in 5 minutes by first tablet, take upto 2 SL tablets at 5 minutes intervals. Take SL tablets 5–15 minutes prior to situation causing pain (sexual intercourse, cold exposure, stress), use paracetamol for headache. Remove patch at bedtime and apply on arising. Avoid alcohol, nitrate; syncope, severe shock like state may occur
- **Desired Outcome:** Decrease in angina and increase in activity tolarance.

1. Isosorbide

Dosage:

- Isosorbide dinitrate: Adults:
  PO: Prevention of angina: 5–20 mg, 2–3 times/day
  SL: Acute attack of angina: 2.5–5 mg, may be repeated every 5–10 minutes for 3 dose in 15–30 minutes. Prophylaxis of angina: 2.5–5 mg SOS
- Isosorbide mononitrate: Adults: PO: 5–20 mg twice daily.

Brands:

- Dinitrate: 5, 10 mg Tab; Sorbitrate. 20, 40 mg Cap; Cardicap
- Mononitrate: 10, 20, 40 mg Tabs; Angitab, Monopark.

2. Nitroglycerine

Dosage:

- Adults: PO: 2.5–9 mg every 8–12 hours
  SL: 0.3–0.6 mg, may be repeated every 5 minutes for 3 doses
  IV: 5 μg/minutes, can be increased slowly up to 20 μg/minutes
  Oint: 1–2 inch every 8 hours (1 inch = 15 mg)
  Patch: 0.1–0.6 mg/hours (Max: 0.8 mg/hour)

- Children: IV: Initial dose of 0.25–0.5 μg/kg/minutes can be increased slowly up to 5 μg/kg/minutes.

Brands: 0.5 mg Tabs; Angised. 2.5, 6.5 mg Cap; NGlong. 5 mg/ml Inj; Nitroject. 5,10 mg patch; Nitroderm TTS. 2% oint; Myovin.

Nursing Consideration: For IV, use glass bottles only and special tubing provided with it. It can be given diluted in D5W/NS to a max concentration of 400 μg/ml.

Chapter

4 Antianxiety Agents

Includes: (A) Benzodiazepines
(B) Selective Serotonin Reuptake Inhibitors (SSRIs)
(C) Miscellaneous

General Nursing Consideration

- **Assess:** CBC, LFT, RFT, platelet and serum electrolytes. BP, HR, respiratory status; level of sedation and anxiety, mental status, sleep pattern periodically
- **Administration:** Chronic therapy may lead to physical and psychological dependence except buspirone. Per Oral (PO) with food. Maintain a quiet, soothing, supervised environment. Keep oxygen and resuscitative equipment ready in event of respiratory depression
- **Advise:** Avoid alcohol and other CNS depressants, activities requiring alertness. Abrupt withdrawal may cause withdrawal symptoms. Advise additional measures; exercise, psychotherapy, relaxation techniques, yoga. Rise slowly to prevent light headedness or fainting. Consume extra fluids and bulk food to mimimize constipating effects
- **Desired Outcome:** Decreased anxiety level.

(A) ANTIANXIETY AGENTS—BENZODIAZEPINES

For action, side effects, details of clobazam, clonazepam, diazepam, lorazepam, midazolam refer to anticonvulsants section (Chapter 10).

Include:
1. Alprazolam
2. Chlordiazepoxide
3. Clobazam
4. Clonazepam
5. Diazepam
6. Flurazepam
7. Lorazepam
8. Midazolam
9. Oxazepam

1. Alprazolam

Uses: Anxiety, panic disorder.

Dosage: Adults: PO

- Anxiety: 0.25–0.5 mg, 2–3 times/day
- Panic disorder: 0.5 mg, 3 times/day

Brands: 0.25, 0.5, 1 mg Tabs; Alpraquil, Alzolam.

Nursing Consideration: To avoid day time sedation administer larger dose at bedtime.

2. Chlordiazepoxide

Uses: Anxiety, alcohol withdrawal, sedation.

Dosage:

- Alcohol withdrawal: Adults: PO: 50–100 mg, may be repeated 2–3 times/day. IM, IV: 50–100 mg, may be repeated in 2–4 hours
- Anxiety: Adults: PO: 5–25 mg 3–4 times/day. IM, IV: 50–100 mg then 25–50 mg as required. Children > 6 years: PO: 5 mg 2–4 times/day. IM, IV: >12 years, 25–50 mg/dose.

Brands: 10, 25 mg Tabs; Cloxide, Librium.

Nursing Consideration: Strictly monitor BP, HR, RR while using parenterally. Prefer IV over IM use. Reconstitute 100 mg in 5 ml of normal saline and administer over 1–2 minutes.

3. Flurazepam

Uses: Anxiety, insomnia.

Dosage: Adults and Children > 15 years: PO: 15–30 mg at bedtime.

Brands: 5, 10 mg Cap; Nindral.

4. Oxazepam

Uses: Anxiety, alcohol withdrawal, sedation.

Dosage: Adults: PO

- Anxiety: 10–30 mg, 3–4 times/day
- Alcohol withdrawal/Sedation: 15–30 mg, 3–4 times/day.

Brands: 15, 30 mg Tabs; Serepax.

(B) ANTIANXIETY AGENTS—SELECTIVE SEROTONIN REUPTAKE INHIBITORS

Refer to antidepressants section (Chapter 11).

(C) ANTIANXIETY AGENTS—MISCELLANEOUS

Include: 1. Buspirone 2. Hydroxyzine 3. Venlafoxine 4. Zolpidem

1. Buspirone

Action: Binds to serotonin and dopamine receptors in the brain.

Uses: Anxiety.

Dosage: Adults: PO: 7.5 mg twice daily (Max: 60 mg/day).

Brands: 5,10 mg Tabs; Buscalm, Buspin.

Side Effects: Nausea, drowsiness, headache, fatigue, blurred vision, rashes, sweating.

2. Hydroxyzine

Action: Antihistaminic, anticholinergic and antiemetic; CNS depressant at the subcortical level.

Uses: Anxiety, sedation, antipruritic, antiemetic.

Dosage:

- Adults: Antianxiety: PO: 25–100 mg, 4 times/day
  Sedation: PO, IM: 50–100 mg single dose
  Vomiting: IM: 25–100 mg every 4–6 hours as needed
  Antipruritic: PO: 25 mg, 3–4 times/day.
- Pediatric: PO: 2 mg/kg/day divided every 4–6 hours. IM: 0.5–1 mg/kg 4–6 hours.

Brands: 10, 25 mg Tabs; 10 mg/5 ml Syp; 6 mg/ml drops; Atarax, Hicope.

Side Effects: Dry mouth, drowsiness, pain at IM site.

3. Venlafoxine

Action: Inhibits norepinephrine and serotonin reuptake in the central nervous system.

Uses: Anxiety, depression.

Dosage: Adults: PO; 75 mg/day in 2–3 divided doses.

Brands: 25, 37.5 and 75 mg Tab; Dalium, Venlift.

Side Effects: Anorexia, AP, constipation, dizziness, headache, seizures, visual disturbances, paresthesia.

4. Zolpidem

Action: Acts by binding to GABA receptors.

Uses: Insomnia, sedation.

Dosage: Adults: PO: 10 mg at bedtime.

Brands: 5, 10 mg Tab; Zanlop, Zolpid.

Side Effects: Anaphylaxis, behavior changes, hallucinations.

* For details of doxepin, trazodone refer to antidepressants chapter.

Chapter 5 Antiarrhythmics

Includes: Class IA to class IV.

These drugs are used to treat and prevent cardiac arrhythmias of various etiology. These are classified from class I to IV.

(A) ANTIARRHYTHMIC—CLASS IA

Includes: 1. Disopyramide 2. Moricizine 3. Procainamide 4. Quinidine Sulfate

Action: Decreases myocardial excitability and conduction velocity.

Side Effects: Nausea, constipation, diarrhea, dry mouth, dizziness, headache, blurred vision, CHF, edema, hypotension, urinary hesitency and retention, agranulocytosis.

General Nursing Consideration

- **Assess:** BP, pulse and ECG throughout therapy; RFT, LFT and serum magnesium, blood glucose, CBC; I/O; daily weight; edema; urinary retention; signs and symptoms of CHF (peripheral edema, JVP, crepts, dyspnea, weight gain)
- **Administration:** Patient should remain supine during IV therapy. IV therapy should be discontinued if; HR <60 or >120/minute, arrhythmia is resolved, PR interval is prolonged, decrease in BP by >15 mm Hg and widening of QRS complex. Teach patient and family members on how to take pulse and immediately report major change in rate. Contraindicated in cardiogenic shock and 1st and IInd degree heart block
- **Advise:** Take exactly as directed even if feeling better. May cause dizziness, avoid activities requiring mental alertness. Avoid extremes of temperature and change position slowly to minimize orthostatic hypotension
- **Desired Outcome:** Decrease or resolution of cardiac arrhythmias.

1. Disopyramide

Uses: Treatment of ventricular tachycardia, uni-or multifocal PVCs, SVTA.

Dosage: Per oral on empty stomach, 1 hour before or 2 hours after meal

- Adults: >50 kg: 150 mg every 6 hourly; <50 kg: 100 mg every 6 hourly
- Children 4–18 years: 6–15 mg/kg/day divided every 6 hourly.
- Infants and children upto 4 years: 10–20 mg/kg/day divided every 6 hourly.

Brands: 100 mg Tab; Regubeat; 10, 150 mg Cap; Norpace.

2. Moricizine

Uses: Treatment of ventricular arrhythmias and tachycardia.

Dosage: Adults (PO): 600–900 mg/day divided 8 hourly.

Brands: 300, 600 mg Tab; Ethmozine.

3. Procainamide

Uses: Treatment of atrial and ventricular premature contraction, ventricular tachycardia, PSVT.

Dosage:

- Adults (IV): 100 mg every 5 minutes until arrhythmia stops
  (IM): 50 mg/kg/day divided every 3–6 hourly
- Children (IV): 3–6 mg/kg/dose over 5 minutes may be repeated every 5–10 minutes as needed. (IM): 20–30 mg/kg/day every 3–6 hourly as needed.

Brands: 100 mg/ml Inj; Pronastyl.

Nursing Consideration: For IV use dilute 100 mg in 10 ml of normal saline (NS) and infuse at the rate of 25 mg/minute. Rapid push may cause asystole and hypotension.

4. Quinidine Sulfate

Uses: Treatment of atrial fibrillation or flutter, ventricular arrhythmias, prevent reccurence of PSVT.

Dosage: PO ± food.

- Adults: 200–400 mg every 4–6 hourly
- Children: 6 mg/kg, 4–5 times/day.

Brands: 100 mg Tab; Natcardine. 200 mg Tab; Quinidine.

Nursing Consideration: Monitor for signs and symptoms of cinchonism (tinnitus, hearing impairment, visual disturbances, nausea, dizziness, headache).

(B) ANTIARRHYTHMIC—CLASS IB

Includes: 1. Lidocaine 2. Mexiletine 3. Phenytoin.

Action: Decreases ERP and APD in cardiac muscle cells.

1. Lidocaine

Uses: Treatment of ventricular tachycardia, fibrillation and ectopy.

Dosage:

- Adults (IV): Initial dose of 1–1.5 mg/kg, may repeat doses of 0.5–0.75 mg/kg every 5–10 minutes if needed to a total dose of 3 mg/kg. Continuous infusion: 1–4 mg/min. ET dose is 2–2.5 of the IV bolus dose.
- Children (IV): 1 mg/kg initial dose, followed by 20–50 μg/kg/min as continuous infusion. ET dose is 2–10 times of IV bolus dose.

Brands: 2% (21.3 mg/ml) Vial; Loxicard, Xylocard.

Side Effects: Common side effects are; nausea, vomiting, bronchospasm, drowsiness, bradycardia, hypotension, blurred vision. Serious side effects are; cardiac arrest, seizures, anaphylaxis.

Nursing Consideration:

- **Assess:** BP, pulse, ECG, serum electrolytes
- **Administration:** For IV use only 1% and 2% solution, give undiluted loading dose over 2–3 minutes followed by continuous infusion. For ET use dilute in 5–10 ml of NS prior to administration followed by 5 manual ventilation. Do not use preservative containing solution for IV use and epinephrine containing solution for arrhythmia. Patient with CHF, acute MI with hypotension, shock, hepatic disease may require dosage reduction to half.

2. Mexiletine

Uses: Treatment and prophylaxis of serious ventricular arrhythmias.

Dosage: PO ± food.

- Adults: 200 mg every 8 hourly. Adjust dosage every 2–3 days
- Children: 1.4–5 mg/kg/dose every 8 hourly. Start with lower doses and increase as required.

Brands: 50 and 100 mg Cap; Mexitil.

Side Effects: Common side effects are; nausea, vomiting, heartburn, tremors, blurred vision, hypotension. Serious side effects are; hepatic necrosis, arrhythmias.

Nursing Consideration: Assess BP, pulse, ECG, CBF, LFT.

3. Phenytoin

Uses: Treatment of ventricular arrhythmias associated with digoxin toxicity, prolonged QT interval and surgical repair of CHD in children.

Dosage:

- Adults (PO): Loading dose of 250 mg, 4 times/day for 1 day, 250 mg twice daily for 2 days then maintenance dose of 300–400 mg/day in 4 divided doses
- Adults and children (IV): Loading dose of 1.25 mg/kg every 5 minutes, may repeat up to total loading dose of 15 mg/kg
- Children (PO, IV): Maintenance dose: 5–10 mg/kg/day divided every 8 hourly.

Brands: 50, 100 Tab; 30 mg/5 ml Syp; 50 mg/ml Inj; Eptoin. 25, 100 mg Cap; 25 mg/5 ml Syp; 50 mg/ml Inj; Dilantin.

Side Effects: Nausea, gingival hyperplasia, ataxia, nystagmus, diplopia, hypotension. Serious side effects are; SJS, agranulocytosis, aplastic anemia.

Nursing Consideration: Assess BP, ECG, respiratory function, CBC, LFT, serum calcium. For IV use dilute in NS in a concentration of 1–10 mg/ml and infuse at the rate of 1–3 mg/kg/min. Maximum rate permitted is 50 mg/min. IV infusion should be followed by NS flushes to avoid local irritation.

(C) ANTIARRHYTHMIC—CLASS IC

Includes: 1. Flecainide 2. Propafenone

Action: Slows conduction in cardiac tissue by altering transport of ions across cell membranes.

Uses: Treatment of ventricular arrhythmias, atrial flutter and fibrillation, PSVT.

Side Effects: Common side effects are; nausea, vomiting, constipation, altered taste, dizziness, conduction disturbances, blurred vision. Serious side effects are; arrhythmias, CHF, chest pain.

General Nursing Consideration

- **Assess:** CBC, RFT, LFT, PT, BP, Pulse, ECG, input and output; daily weight; signs and symptoms of CHF
- **Administration:** PO ± food. Therapy should be initiated in a ICCU setting. Full effect may take 3–5 days to appear
- **Advise:** Take exactly as advised. Gradual dose reduction is recommended. May cause dizziness and visual disturbances.

1. Flecainide

Dosage: PO

- Adults: Life-threatening ventricular arrhythmias: Initially 100 mg 12 hourly and then can be increased every 4 days by 100 mg/kg (Max: 400 mg/day).
- PSVT/AF: Initially 50 mg 12 hourly (Max: 300 mg/day)
- Children: Initially 1–3 mg/kg/day divided every 8 hourly (Max: 8 mg/kg/day).

Brands: 50, 100, 150 mg Tab; Tonpour

Nursing Consideration: Therapy should be discontinued if bone marrow suppression occurs

2. Propafenone

Dosage: Adults (PO): 150 mg every 8 hourly and then can be increased gradually every 3–4 days to 300 mg every 8 hours.

Brands: 150 mg Tab; Rhythmonorm.

(D) ANTIARRHYTHMIC—CLASS II

Includes: 1. Esmolol 2. Propranolol 3. Sotalol

Action: Blocks stimulation of Beta-1 (myocardial) adrenergic receptors. For details of side effects and nursing consideration refer to antianginals—beta-blockers (Chapter 3).

1. Esmolol

Uses: Treatment of sinus and supraventricular tachycardia.

Dosage: IV

- Adults: Loading dose of 500 µg/kg over 1 minute followed by 50 µg/kg/min for 4 minutes. If no response repeat the loading dose and increase further doses by 100 µg/kg/min for 4 minutes (Max: 200 µg/kg/min).
- Children: 50 µg/kg/min, can be increased every 10 minutes to 300 µg/kg/min.

Brands: 10 mg/ml Inj; Cardesmo, Neotach.

Nursing Consideration: IV doses are given in a concentration of 10–20 mg/ml and infused over 1 minute, discontinue or decrease rate if fall in BP or CHF occur.

2. Propranolol

For details refer antianginals: beta-blockers (Chapter 3).

3. Sotalol

Uses: Treatment of ventricular arrhythmia, atrial fibrillation and flutter.

Dosage: Adults (PO): 80 mg twice daily, can be increased gradually up to 160 mg/day in 2–3 divided doses.

Brands: 40 and 80 mg Tab; Sotagard.

Nursing Consideration: PO given on empty stomach, 1 hour before or 2 hours after meals. Its use should be avoid along with antacids containing aluminium and magnesium salts within 2 hours.

(E) ANTIARRHYTHMIC—CLASS III

Includes: Amiodarone.

Action: Prolongs ERP and APD in myocardial tissue.

Uses: PO: Ventricular arrhythmias unresponsive to other therapy. IV: Ventricular fibrillation and tachycardia in patients not able to take PO therapy.

Dosage:

- Ventricular arrhythmias:
  Adults (PO): 800–1600 mg/day divided 12 hourly for 1–3 weeks, then 600–800 mg/day divided 12 hourly for 1 month, then 400 mg/day maintenance dose. (IV): 150 mg over 10 minutes followed by 360 mg given over 6 hours, then 540 mg over next 18 hours. Then continue at the rate of 0.5 mg/min till it can be given orally.
  Infants and children (PO): 10 mg/kg/day for 10 days, then 5 mg/kg/day once daily for several weeks, then taper off to 2.5 mg/kg/day. (IV): 5 mg/kg loading dose over 20–60 minutes, may be repeated to maximum dose of 15 mg/kg/day
- Supraventricular tachycardia (PO):
  Adults: 600–800 mg/day for 1 week, then 400 mg/day for 3–8 weeks then maintenance dose of 200–400 mg/day.
  Children: Same as given for ventricular arrhythmia PO doses.

Brands: 100 and 200 mg Tab; 50 mg/ml Inj; Cardarone, Eurythmic, Ritebeat.

Side Effects: Common side effects are; nausea, vomiting, anorexia, constipation, dizziness, ataxia, paresthesia, tremors, poor coordination, hypotension, bradycardia. Serious side effects are; ARDS, CHF, Pulmonary toxicity, liver dysfunction, toxic epidermal necrosis.

Nursing Consideration:

- **Assess:** LFT, thyroid function; ECG, BP, pulse, CXR, assess pulmonary status, symptoms of ARDS, neurotoxicity, ophthalmic examination
- **Administration:** PO ± meals. Hypomagnesemia and hypokalemia should be corrected prior to therapy. For IV use dilute in D5W to achieve a concentration of 1.5 mg/ml and infuse over 10 minutes. Avoid using IV doses for >96 hours
- **Advise:** Teach how to monitor pulse and BP. Bluish discoloration of face, neck and arms may occur. Advise to take exactly as directed.

(F) ANTIARRHYTHMIC—CLASS IV

Includes: 1. Diltiazem
2. Verapamil

For details refer to antianginals—calcium channel blockers (Chapter 3).

(G) ANTIARRHYTHMIC—MISCELLANEOUS

Includes: Adenosine

Action: Slows conduction through AV node.

Uses: Treatment of PSVT, supraventricular tachycardia.

Dosage: IV

- Adults and children >50 kg: 6 mg stat, if no response within 1-2 minutes then 12 mg may be given; may be repeated 12 mg bolus if needed
- Children <50 kg: 0.05-0.1 mg/kg as a rapid bolus, if no response within 1-2 minutes then increase dose by 0.05-0.1 mg/kg until PSVT terminated or maximum dose of 0.3 mg/kg is reached.

Brands: 3 mg/ml Inj; Adenocor, Adenoject.

Side Effects: Metallic taste, dizziness, headache, blurred vision, dyspnea, hyperventilation, flushing, arrhythmias, bradycardia, chest pain.

Nursing Consideraton:

- **Assess:** BP, Pulse, ECG, respiratory status
- **Administration:** Given undiluted in a concentration of 3 mg/ml over 1-2 seconds via peripheral line as proximal to trunk as possible. IV administration into lower extremities may result in therapeutic failure or requirement of higher doses. Slow administration may cause increase in HR. Follow each dose with NS flush (20 ml in adults and 5-10 ml in infants and children)
- **Advise:** Change position slowly to avoid orthostatic hypotension. Dose higher than 12 mg may cause hypotension.

Chapter

6 Antiasthmatics

Includes: A. Adrenergics
B. Anticholinergics
C. Corticosteroids
D. Leukotriene antagonists
E. Mast cell stabilizers
F. Xanthines

(A) ANTIASTHMATICS—ADRENERGICS

Includes: 1. Albuterol/Salbutamol
2. Bambuterol
3. Epinephrine/Adrenaline
4. Formoterol
5. Levosalbutamol
6. Salmeterol
7. Terbutaline

Action: They act by increasing intracellular cAMP production at β-adrenergic receptors which leads to bronchodilation. Epinephrine in addition also has α-adrenergic agonist effect.

Side Effects: Common side effects are; nervousness, restlessness, tremors, palpitation, arrhythmias, HT, tachycardia. Serious side effects are; paradoxical bronchospasm and anaphylaxis.

General Nursing Considerations

- **Assess:** BP, pulse, respiratory pattern, lung sounds, type of secretions, PFT, paradoxical bronchospasm, chest pain, cardiovascular status, ECG
- **Administration:** Teach technique of nebulization, MDI use, how to use spacer in children. Give it round the clock to maintain therapeutic plasma levels. Do not refrigerate inhaler, shake it well before use; prime it before first use by releasing 2–4 sprays into the air. Use spacer device with inhaler for children <8 years of age. Long-acting adrenergics should not be used during acute attack of asthma
- **Advise:** Take exactly as directed. Avoid exposure to smoking, perfumes, dust and other respiratory irritants. Maintain fluid intake of 1500–2000 mL/day to decrease viscosity of airway secretions. If on multidrug therapy, use bronchodilator first and 5 minutes gap should be there before administering other medications. Rinse mouth with water after each inhalation to minimize dry mouth and throat. Report immediately if diaphoresis, dizziness, palpitation or chest pain occur. Avoid getting aerosol in eyes. Regular consistent use is essential for maximum benefit, but overuse may result in reduced effectiveness, paradoxical reaction and death from cardiac arrest.

- **Desired Outcome:** Increased ease of breathing; prevention or reduction in symptoms of asthma; reduction in frequency of asthma attack; prevention of exercise induced asthma; as applicable to particular drug.

1. Albuterol/Salbutamol

Uses: Short and long-term control of asthma, prevention of exercise induced asthma.

Dosage:

- Acute asthma attacks:
  Nebulization: Adults: 2.5–5 mg every 20 minutes for 3 doses then 2.5–10 mg every 1–4 hourly as needed
  Children: 0.15 mg/kg (Min: 2.5 mg) every 20 min for 3 doses then 0.15–0.3 mg/kg (Max: 10 mg) every 2–4 hours as needed
  Inhalation: 100 μg/spray
  Adults: 4–8 puff every 20 minutes for 3 doses then as needed
  Children: 4–8 puff every 20 minutes for 3 doses then as needed
- Maintenance therapy:
  PO: Adults and children ≥ 12 years: 2–4 mg/dose 3–4 times/day
  Children 6-12 years: 2 mg/dose 3–4 times/day
  Children 2–6 years: 0.1–0.2 mg/kg/dose, 3 times/day
  Inhalation: Adults and children ≥ 4 years: 1–2 puff 4–6 hourly
- Exercise induced asthma: 2 puff 5–30 minutes before exercise.

Brands: 2 and 4 mg Tab; 2 mg/5 ml Syp; 2.5 mg respules, 200 and 400 μg rotacaps; Asthalin. 100 μg/puff MDI; Salbair. Also available in combinations.

Nursing Consideration: PO + food to decrease GI discomfort. 1–2 mg/ml solution do not require dilution.

2. Bambuterol

Uses: Long-term control of asthma, chronic bronchitis.

Dosage: PO:

- Adults: 10–20 mg OD
- Children: 6–12 years; 10 mg OD. 2–5 years; 5 mg OD.

Brands: 10, 20 mg Tab; 1 mg/ml Syp; Bambudil, Roburol.

3. Epinephrine/Adrenaline

Uses: Bronchospasm, anaphylactic reaction, cardiac arrest.

Dosage:

- Adults: Asystole
  IV: 1 mg every 3–5 minutes
  Intratracheal: 2–2.5 mg
  IM, SC: 0.1–0.5 mg every 10–15 minutes
  Continuous IV Infusion: Initial 1 μg/min, then titrate to desired effect.
- Infants and Children:
  IM: <30 kg, 0.15 mg; >30 kg, 0.3 mg
  SC: 0.01 mg/kg (0.01 ml/kg/dose of 1:1000 solution). Max: 0.5 mg

- Bradycardia: It can be repeated as needed
  IV: 0.01 mg/kg (0.1 ml/kg of 1:10,000 solution). Max: 1 mg
  Intratracheal: 0.1 mg/kg (0.1 ml/kg of 1:1000 solution).
- Asystole or pulseless arrest: It may be repeated as needed.
  IV: 0.01 mg/kg (0.1 ml/kg of 1:10,000 solution)
  Intratracheal: 0.1 mg/kg (0.1 ml/kg of 1:1000 solution)
- Nebulization: 0.25–0.5 ml of 2.25% racemic epinephrine diluted in 3 ml of normal saline(NS).

Brands: 1 mg/ml Inj; Vasocon.

Nursing Consideration: Monitor BP, pulse, respiration and ECG during IV use. Assess for volume status and correct hypovolemia before giving it IV. Avoid IM injection in gluteal muscle. Each IV dose should be followed by 20 mL of saline flush and each intratracheal dose should be followed by several positive pressure ventilations. Nebulization and intratracheal dose should be given diluted in 3–5 ml of NS.

4. Formoterol

Uses: Long-term maintenance treatment of asthma and COPD, prevention of exercise induced asthma.

Dosage:
- Bronchodilation (asthma/COPD):
  Adults and Children ≥5 years (Inhalation): 12 µg BD
- Prevention of exercise induced asthma:
  Adults and Children ≥5 years (Inhalation): 12 µg, 15 minutes prior to exercise.

Brands: 12 µg inhaler and rotacaps; Foratec. Also available in combination.

5. Levosalbutamol

Uses: Short-term control of bronchospasm.

Dosage: Nebulization.
- Adults and Children >12 years: 0.63–1.25 mg, 3 times/day
- Children 6–11 years: 0.31 mg, 3 times/day
- Children 2–6 years: 0.16 mg, 3 times/day.

Brands: 0.63 and 1.25 mg/2.5 ml respulse; 100 µg rotacap; Levolin.

6. Salmeterol

Uses: Long-term treatment of asthma and COPD, prevention of exercise induced asthma.

Dosage: Adults and Children ≥5 years. (Inhalation): 50 µg BD. For exercise induced asthma, give 30 minutes prior.

Brands: 20 µg Salbutamol+125 µg Fluticasone/puff; Esiflo-125, Vent-SF. 50 µg Salbutamol + 100 µg Fluticasone, Rotacaps; Esiflo-100, Seroflo.

7. Terbutaline

Uses: Long and short-term control of reversible airway obstruction (asthma, COPD, emphysema).

Dosage:

- Adults and Children ≥12 years: PO: 2.5–5 mg/dose 6–8 hourly
  SC: 0.25 mg/dose can be repeated every 20 minutes × 3 doses
- Children <12 years: PO: 0.05 mg/kg/dose every 8 hourly (Max: 5 mg/day)
  SC: 0.005–0.01 mg/kg/dose every 20 minutes × 3 doses
- Nebulization: Adults and Children: 0.01–0.03 mg/kg (Min: 0.1 mg/dose) 4–6 hourly.

Brands: 2.5 and 5 Tab; 1.5 mg/5 ml Syp; 0.5 mg/ml Inj; 0.25 mg/puff inhaler; Bricanyl.

Nursing Consideration: PO + food. Give SC at lateral deltoid muscle.

(B) ANTIASTHMATICS—ANTICHOLINERGICS

Includes: 1. Ipratropium 2. Tiotropium

Actions: Acts by decreasing intracellular levels of cGMP leading to bronchodilation.

Nursing Consideration: Refer adrenergics (Page No. 29).

1. Ipratropium

Uses: Long-term control of bronchospasm (asthma, COPD, bronchitis).

Dosage:

- Adults and Children ≥12 years: Nebulization: 250 μg 6 hourly
  Inhaler: 40–80 μg, 6 hourly
- Children 4–12 years: Nebulization: 125–250 μg, 3 times/day
  Inhaler: 20–40 μg, 6 hourly

Brands: 500 μg/2.5 ml respule, 40 μg rotacaps, 20 μg/puff inhaler; Ipravent.

Side Effects: Headache, dizziness, blurred vision, hypotension, palpitation, GI discomfort.

Nursing Consideration: Nebulization solution should be diluted in 2–4 ml of NS.

2. Tiotropium

Uses: Long-term control of bronchospasm.

Dosage: Adults (Inhalation): 18 μg OD.

Brands: 8 μg/puff Inhaler; 18 μg rotacaps; Tiate, Tiova.

Side Effects: Common side effects are dry mouth and palpitation. Serious one is angioedema.

(C) ANTIASTHMATICS—CORTICOSTEROIDS

Includes: 1. Beclomethasone 2. Betamethasone
3. Budesonide 4. Ciclesonide
5. Dexamethasone 6. Fluticasone
7. Hydrocortisone 8. Methylprednisolone
9. Prednisolone 10. Triamcinolone

Action: These agents are either locally or systemic acting anti-inflammatory and immune modifier (1, 3, 4 and 6 are local acting and rest are systemic acting).

Side Effects: For systemic acting drugs: Common side effects are; nausea, vomiting, anorexia, adrenal suppression, acne, decreased wound healing, ecchymosis, increased skin fragility, hirsutism, headache, depression, HT, osteoporosis, muscles weakness, cushingoid appearance. Serious side effects are; peptic ulceration and thromboembolism.

For local acting: Common side effects are; diarrhea, dry mouth, esophageal candidiasis, taste disturbances, headache, cataracts, dysphonia, hoarseness, adrenal suppression. Serious one is Churg-Strauss syndrome.

General Nursing Consideration

- **Assess:** Blood glucose, serum electrolyte, BP, ECG, input and output, daily weight; peripheral edema, dyspnea, mucous membranes for signs of fungal infection; signs of adrenal insufficiency (anorexia, nausea, weakness, fatigue, hypotension, hypoglycemia, weight loss); withdrawal symptoms (muscle and joint pain, depression, lassitude). Monitor growth rate in children on chronic therapy
- **Administration:** Use lowest effective dose and keep 1–2 minutes gap between inhalation. Avoid allergy test during steroid therapy. Systemic steroids should be administered in the morning to coincide with the body's normal secretion of cortisol. PO with meal to decrease GI discomfort
- **Advise:** Take exactly as directed. Always taper off. Notify sore throat or sore mouth. Avoid exposing eyes to inhalation steroids and wash face after inhalation. Avoid vaccination during systemic steroid use. Rinse mouth after inhalation to decrease chances of oral candidiasis. Take diet rich in protein, calcium, Vitamin-A, B, C, D, folate; zinc, potassium and low in carbohydrate and sodium. Use with extra caution in patient with respiratory TB, untreated systemic infection. To prevent and relieve epigastric pain take antacids 3–4 times per day
- **Desired Outcome:** Improvement in symptoms of asthma; decrease in inflammation, allergic reaction, autoimmune disorder as applicable to particular drug.

1. Beclomethasone

Uses: Long-term control of asthma.

Dosage: Adults and Children ≥12 years: 40–60 μg BD (Max: 320 μg BD). Children 5–11 years: 40 μg BD (Max: 80 μg BD).

Brands: 40, 50, 100, 200, 250 μg/puff inhaler; Beclate. 100, 200, 400 μg rotacaps; Beclate.

2. Betamethasone

Uses: Anti-inflammatory, immunosuppressant, corticosteroid replacement therapy.

Dosage:

- PO: Adults: 0.6–7.2 mg/day in single or divided doses
  Children: 0.0175–0.25 mg/kg/day divided 8 hourly
- IM: Adults: 0.6–9 mg/day divided 12 hourly
  Children: 0.0175–0.25 mg/kg/day divided 8 hourly

Brands: 0.5 and 1 mg Tab; 0.5 mg/ml drops; 4 mg/ml Inj; Betnesol, Stemin.

3. Budesonide

Uses: Long-term control of asthma.

Dosage: Adults: 200–800 μg BD. Children ≥6 years 200–400 μg BD.

Brands: 0.25, 0.5 and 1 mg respules; 100 and 200 μg inhaler; 100, 200 and 400 μg rotacaps; Budecort.

4. Ciclesonide

Uses: Long-term control of asthma.

Dosage: Adults and Children ≥12 years (Inhalation): 80–160 μg OD in the evening.

Brands: 80 μg rotacaps; Ciclohale.

5. Dexamethasone

Uses: Anti-inflammatory, airway edema, antiemetic, bacterial meningitis, cerebral edema, BPD.

Dosage:

- Anti-inflammatory (PO, IM, IV):
  Adults: 0.75–9 mg/day divided 6–12 hourly
  Children: 0.08–0.3 mg/kg/day divided 6–12 hourly
- Airway edema:
  Adults and Children (PO, IM, IV): 0.5–2 mg/kg/day divided 6 hourly
  Neonates (IV): 0.25–1 mg/kg/dose for 1–3 doses
- Cerebral Edema:
  Adults: Initially 10 mg IV, then 4 mg IM/IV 12 hourly until desired response then PO, taper over 5–7 days
  Children (PO, IM, IV): Initially 1–2 mg/kg as a single dose. Maintenance, 1–1.5 mg/kg/day in divided doses (Max. dose: 16 mg/day)

- Bacterial meningitis: Children >2 months (IV): 0.6 mg/kg/day divided 6 hourly for the first 4 days of antibiotic therapy
- Antiemetic (chemotherapy induced), IV: Initial 10 mg/m^2/dose (Max: 20 mg) then 5 mg/m^2/dose 6 hourly
- BPD: Neonate (PO, IV): 0.5–0.6 mg/kg/day divided 12 hourly for 3–7 days, then taper off gradually.

Brands: 0.5 mg Tab; 4 mg/ml Inj; 0.5 mg/ml drops; Decdon, Dexona.

Nursing Consideration: Dose <10 mg can be given undiluted IV slowly but high doses must be diluted in D_5W or NS and given over 15–30 minutes.

6. Fluticasone

Uses: Long-term control of asthma.

Dosage: Adults and Children >12 years: 88–440 μg twice daily. Children 4–11 years: 88 μg twice daily.

Brands: 25, 50 and 125 μg/puff inhaler; 50, 100, 250 μg rotacaps; 0.5 and 2 mg respules; Flohale.

7. Hydrocortisone

Uses: Anti-inflammatory/immunosuppressive, status asthmaticus, shock, adrenocortical insufficiency.

Dosage:

- Status asthmaticus: Adults (IV): 100–500 mg 6 hourly
  Children (IV): Initial 4–8 mg/kg (Max: 250 mg) then 2 mg/kg/dose 6 hourly
- Anti-inflammatory/Immunosuppressive:
  Adults (PO, IV, IM): 15–240 mg 12 hourly.
  Infants and Children (PO): 2.5–10 mg/kg/day in divided doses
  (IM, IV): 1–5 mg/kg/day divided 12 hourly
- Shock: Adults (IV): 500 mg every 2–6 hourly
  Children (IV): 50 mg/kg then repeated as required
- Acute adrenal insufficiency:
  Adults: Initially 100 mg IV bolus then 300 mg/day in divided doses 8 hourly, titrate further doses.
  Children: Initially 1–2 mg/kg/dose IV bolus then 25–150 mg/day in divided doses 6–8 hourly.

Brands:100 mg vial; Efcorlin, Unicort. 200 mg vial; Primacort.

Nursing Consideration: IV bolus is given in a concentration of 50 mg/ml over 3–5 minutes and infusion at 1 mg/ml over 20–30 minutes.

8. Methylprednisolone

Uses: Status asthmaticus, anti-inflammatory/immunosuppressive, acute spinal cord injury.

Dosage:

- Status asthmaticus: Adults: (PO, IV): 120–180 mg/day divided doses for 48 hours then 60–80 mg/day in divided doses.
  Children (IV): 2 mg/kg/dose, then 0.5–1 mg/kg/dose 6 hourly

- Anti-inflammatory/Immunosuppressive:
  Adults (IM, IV): 40–250 mg 4–6 hourly
  Children (PO, IM, IV): 0.5–1.7 mg/kg/day in divided doses
  Pulse therapy: 15–30 mg/kg/dose, given over 30 minutes once daily for 3 days
- Acute spinal cord injury (IV): 30 mg/kg over 15 minutes followed 15 minutes later by a continuous infusion of 5 mg/kg/hr for 23 hours.

Brands: 4 and 16 mg Tab; Mypred, Zempred. 40, 125, 500 mg and 1 g vial; MPSS, Premisol.

9. Prednisolone

Uses: Acute asthma, anti-inflammatory/immunosuppressive, nephrotic syndrome and variety of endocrine, rheumatic, collagen, allergic, hematologic diseases.

Dosage: PO

- Adults: Most uses: 5–60 mg/day in single or divided doses.
  Asthma: 120–180 mg/day in divided doses for 48 hours then 60–80 mg/day in 2 divided doses
- Children: Anti-inflammatory/immunosuppressive: 0.1–2 mg/kg/day in 1–4 divided doses.
  Nephrotic syndrome: 2 mg/kg/day in 1–3 divided doses (Max: 80 mg/day) until urine is protein free for 4–6 weeks, followed by 2 mg/kg/dose every other day in the morning, gradually taper off over 4–6 weeks
  Asthma: 1 mg/kg 6 hourly for 48 hours then 1–2 mg/kg/day (Max: 60 mg/day) divided 12 hourly.

Brands: 5, 10, 20 and 40 mg Tab; Pensone, Wysolone. 10 mg/5 ml Syp; Kidpred. 20, 30 and 40 mg Vial; Anesolin.

10. Triamcinolone

Uses: Various anti-inflammatory and immunosuppressive condition.

Dosage: Adults (IM): 40–80 mg every 4 weeks. Children (IM): 40 mg every 4 weeks.

Intra-articular, intrabursal or tendon sheath injection:

Adults and Children ≥12 years: 2–20 mg every 3–4 weeks. Children 6 to <12 years: 2.5–15 mg every 3–4 weeks.

PO: Adults and Children >12 years: 4–100 mg/day in divided doses.

Brands: 4 mg Tab; 10 and 40 mg Inj; Kenacort, Tricort.

(D) ANTIASTHMATICS—LEUKOTRIENE ANTAGONISTS

Includes: 1. Montelukast 2. Zafirlukast 3. Zileuton

Action: Antagonizes the effects of leukotrienes resulting in decrease in bronchospasm, mucosal edema and mucus production.

Uses: Prophylaxis and long-term treatment of asthma; montelukast in addition also used for severe allergic rhinitis.

Side Effects: GI discomfort, raised liver enzymes, fatigue, headache, arthralgia, myalgia.

Nursing Consideration: These agents are not indicated for acute attack of asthma. Take regularly as advised. Desired effects are prevention or reduction in symptoms of asthma and decrease in severity of allergic rhinitis. Continue other antiasthmatic medications as prescribed. Avoid triggers i.e. dust, chemicals, smoking, pollutants, pets and perfumes.

1. Montelukast

Dosage: Give daily in the evening for asthma and, for allergy it can be given at any time of the day, give with meals.

- Adults and Children ≥4 years: 10 mg OD
- Children: 6–14 years: 5 mg OD. 2–5 years: 4 mg OD. 6–23 months: 4 mg OD.

Brands: 4, 5 and 10 mg Tab; Emlucast, Montelast.

2. Zafirlukast

Dosage: Give orally at regular intervals on an empty stomach 1 hour before or 2 hours after meals. Avoid in liver dysfunction.

- Adults and Children ≥12 years: 20 mg BD
- Children, 5–11 years: 10 mg BD.

Brands: 10, 20 mg Tab; Zuvair.

3. Zileuton

Dosage: PO ± food. Adults and Children >12 years: 600 mg, 4 times/day.

Brands: 600 mg Tab; Zyflo.

(E) ANTIASTHMATICS—MAST CELL STABILIZERS

Includes: 1. Nedocromil 2. Sodium Cromoglycate

Action: Prevents mast cell release of histamines, leukotrienes and SRS-A.

Uses: For long-term control of asthma, prevention of exercise induced asthma. Cromoglycate in addition is also used for prevention and treatment of allergic rhinitis.

Nursing Consideration:

- **Assess:** Respiratory status, triggering factors, PFT, CXR
- **Administration:** Use bronchodilator and steroids if required
- **Advise:** Start after acute episode is over.

1. Nedocromil

Dosage: Adults and Children ≥6 years (Inhalation): 1.75 mg/puff up to 2 inhalations 4 times/day.

Brands: 1.75 mg/puff inhaler; Alocril.

2. Sodium Cromoglycate

Dosage:

- PO: Adults and Children ≥12 years: 200 mg, 4 times/day.
  Children: 2–12 years:100 mg, 4 times/day
- Intranasal: Adults and Children ≥2 years: 2 spray in each nostril 3 times/day
- Inhalation:
  Nebulization: Adults and Children ≥2 years: 20 mg upto 4 times/day.
  Inhaler: Adults and Children ≥12 years: 800–1600 μg upto 4 times/day.
  Children 5–12 years: 800 μg upto 2–3 times/day.

Brands: 5 mg/puff inhaler; 10 mg/2 ml respules; 20 mg rotacaps; Cromal. 2% nasal spray; Ifiral.

(F) ANTIASTHMATICS—XANTHINES

Includes: 1. Aminophylline 2. Doxophylline 3. Theophylline

Action: Acts by increasing intracellular level of cAMP which causes bronchodilation, increases force of diaphragmatic contractility.

Uses: Bronchodilation (asthma, COPD), to increase diaphragmatic contractility, apnea of prematurity (aminophylline).

Side Effects: Serious side effects are seizures, arrhythmias. Most common side effects are anxiety, nausea, vomiting, tachycardia.

Nursing Consideration: Also refer to adrenergics—nursing considerations for administration precautions (Page No. 29). Loading dose should be decreased or eliminated if theophylline preparation has been used in preceding 24 hours. Aminophylline is 80% of theophylline (100 mg aminophylline = 80 mg theophylline). Wait to initiate PO therapy for at least 4–6 hours after switching from IV therapy.

1. Aminophylline

Dosage: IV

- Adults, children and infants: Acute bronchospasm: Loading dose of 6 mg/kg given over 20–30 minutes. Followed by maintenance dose as follows:
  Adults and Children >12 years: 0.7 mg/kg/hr
  9–12 years: 0.9 mg/kg/hr
  1–9 years: 1–1.2 mg/kg/hr
  6 months–1 years: 0.6–0.7 mg/kg/hr
  6 weeks–6 months: 0.5 mg/kg/hr

  Intermittent doses can be determined as follows:

$$\frac{\text{Hourly infusion rate} \times 24 \text{ hr}}{\text{Desired no.of doses/day}}$$

- Apnea of prematurity (IV): Loading dose of 5 mg/kg followed by maintenance dose of 5 mg/kg/day divided 12 hourly.

Brands: 100 mg Tab; 25 mg/ml Inj; Aminophylline.

Nursing Consideration: For IV dilute in NS/D_5W/D_{10}W/RL to a concentration of 1 mg/ml and infuse over 20–30 minutes (Max concentration: 25 mg/ml and maximum rate is 25 mg/min in adults and 0.36 mg/kg/min in children).

2. Doxophylline

Uses: Bronchospasm (bronchial asthma and COPD).

Dosage: Adults (PO): 400 mg BD. Children >6 years: 12 mg/kg/day divided 12 hourly.

Brands: 400 mg Tab; Doxobid, Doxovent. 100 mg/5 ml Syp; Synasma.

3. Theophylline

Dosage: PO + food.

- Acute bronchospasm: Adults, children and infants: Loading dose of 5 mg/kg followed by maintenance dose as follows;
  Adults: 10 mg/kg/day divided 8 hourly
  12–16 years: 13 mg/kg/day divided 8 hourly
  9–12 years: 16 mg/kg/day divided 8 hourly
  1–9 years: 20–24 mg/kg/day divided 8 hourly
  6 months–1 year: 12–18 mg/kg/day divided 8 hourly
  6 weeks–6 months: 10 mg/kg/day divided 8 hourly.
- Apnea of prematurity: Neonates: Loading dose is 4 mg/kg/dose.

Brands: 200 mg Tab; Phylobid. 400 and 600 mg Tab; Phloday, Theoday. 80 mg/ml elixir; Broncodril.

Chapter 7

Antibiotics

Includes: (A) Aminoglycosides (B) Carbapenems (C) Cephalosporins (D) Fluoroquinolones (E) Imidazoles (F) Macrolides (G) Penicillins (H) Tetracyclines (I) Miscellaneous

(A) ANTIBIOTICS—AMINOGLYCOSIDES

Include: 1. Amikacin 2. Gentamicin 3. Kanamycin 4. Neomycin 5. Streptomycin 6. Tobramycin

Action: Inhibits protein synthesis in susceptible bacteria by binding to ribosomal subunits.

Side Effects: Common side effects are; nausea, vomiting, ataxia, vertigo, ototoxicity, nephrotoxicity, neuromuscular blockade, tremors, muscle weakness, convulsions.

General Nursing Considerations

- **Assess:** RFT, LFT, urine, signs and symptoms of infection (vitals, CBC, wound condition, urine, stool, sputum), input and output and daily weight for hydration and renal status. Signs of superinfection (fever, diarrhea, vaginal discharge, stomatitis, respiratory infection, increased weakness). Assess hearing and vestibular dysfunction, neurological status in CNS cases
- **Administration:** Discontinue drug at first sign of hearing loss or tinnitus. Maintain good hydration (1.5–2 L/day intake). Use with caution in renal and hearing impairment, neuromuscular disease. Flush IV line with normal saline (NS) after drug infusion. Avoid co-administration with penicillins and cephalosporins and keep a gap of 1 hour between their infusion. Give IM deep into a well developed muscle and rotate site. Administer for only 7–10 days
- **Advise:** Drink plenty of fluid. Report the following immediately (hearing loss, tinnitus, vertigo, difficult micturition)
- **Desired Outcome:** Resolution of signs and symptoms of infection, e.g. prevention of infection in intestinal surgery, improved neurological status in hepatic encephalopathy, endocarditis prophylaxis; as applicable to a particular drug.

1. Amikacin

Uses: Gram negative enteric infections; documented mycobacterial infection susceptible to amikacin.

Dosage: IM, IV

- Adults and children: 15 mg/kg/day divided every 8–12 hourly (Max: 1.5 g/day)
- Term neonates: 7.5–10 mg/kg/day divided every 12 hourly.

Brands: 100, 250, 500 mg Vial; Amicin, Amikef, Mikacin.

Nursing Consideration: IV doses are given diluted in D5W/NS/RL in a maximum concentration of 10 mg/mL and infuse over 30 minutes.

2. Gentamicin

Uses: CNS, bone, RTI, SSTI, UTI, septicemia; infective endocarditis prophylaxis; gram negative and some gram positive *Staphylococcus.*

Dosage: IM, IV.

- Adults: Usual dosage: 3–6 mg/kg/day divided every 8 hourly
  Endocarditis prophylaxis: 1.5 mg/kg within 30 minutes of starting procedure along with ampicillin or vancomycin
- Infants and children: 2–2.5 mg/kg/dose every 8 hourly
  Endocarditis prophylaxis: Same as above.

Brands: 10 and 40 mg/ml Vial; Biogaracin, Genticyn, G-Mycin.

Nursing Consideration: IV doses are given diluted in NS/RL/D_5W in a concentration of 10 mg/ml and infused over ½–2 hours.

3. Kanamycin

Uses: Gram negative infection; also active against staphylococci, CNS, RTI, UTI, GUTI, SSTI; *Mycobacterium tuberculosis* infection.

Dosage: IM, IV.

Adults and children: 5 mg/kg every 8 hours.

Brands: 500, 750 and 1000 mg Vial; Kanamac, kancin.

Nursing Consideration: For IV use dilute 500 mg in 100–200 ml of NS/RL/D_5W in a concentration of 2.5–5 mg/ml and infuse over 30–60 minutes.

4. Neomycin

Uses: To prepare GIT before surgery, treatment of hepatic encephalopathy and diarrhea caused by *E. coli.*

Dosage: PO+food.

- Adults: 500–2000 mg every 6–8 hours
- Children: 50–100 mg/kg/day divided every 6–8 hours.

Brands: 350 mg Cap; Neomycin sulfate.

Nursing Consideration: For preoperative bowel antisepsis more frequent dosing schedule is used along with erythromycin, a low residue diet and enema.

5. Streptomycin

For details refer to antituberculars (Chapter 26).

6. Tobramycin

Uses: Treatment of gram negative infection including *P. aeruginosa*; LRTI, UTI, septicemia, abdominal and orthopedic infections.

Dosage: IM, IV.

- Adults: 3–6 mg/kg/day divided every 8 hours
- Children: 2–2.5 mg/kg/dose every 8 hours.

Brands: 20, 60, 80 mg Vial; Tobacin, Tobax, Tobraneg.

Nursing Consideration: IV doses given diluted in 50–100 ml of D5W/RL/NS in a concentration of 10 mg/ml and infuse over 30–60 min.

(B) ANTIBIOTICS—CARBAPENEMS

Includes: 1. Imipenem/Cilastatin 2. Meropenem

Action: These agents acts by binding to bacterial cell wall resulting in cell death.

Side Effects: Common side effects are; nausea, vomiting, rash, dizziness. Serious side effects are; seizures, anaphylaxis, pseudomembranous colitis, apnea, hepatitis.

General Nursing Considerations

- **Assess:** CBC, RFT, LFT; Vitals; culture and sensitivity, signs and symptoms of infection and anaphylaxis
- **Administration:** May cause dizziness avoid activities requiring mental alertness. Report immediately for signs and symptoms of superinfection, allergy and diarrhea
- **Desired Outcome:** Resolution of signs and symptoms of infection.

1. Imipenem/Cilastatin

Combination of imipenem with cilastatin prevents its renal inactivation resulting in higher urinary concentration.

Uses: Treatment of LRTI, UTI, SSTI, bone and joint; septicemia and endocarditis.

Dosage: IM, IV.

- Adults: Serious infection: 500–1000 mg every 6–8 hours
  Mild to moderate infection: 250–500 mg every 6 hours
- Infants ≥ 3 months and children: 15–25 mg/kg every 6 hours
  Infants 4 weeks – 3 months: 25 mg/kg every 6 hours
- Neonates < 4 weeks: 25 mg/kg every 6–8 hours.

Brands: Imipenem + Cilastatin: 500+500 and 250+250 mg; Cimispect, IME- CILA.

Nursing Consideration: IV doses given diluted in 10 ml of D_5W/NS and this is further diluted to 100 ml in a concentration of 2.5–5 mg/mL and infused over 15–30 minutes. Rapid infusion may cause nausea and vomiting, if these occur then decrease infusion rate. Avoid IV use in children with CNS infections due to the risk of seizures and in children with impaired renal function.

2. Meropenem

Uses: Treatment of meningitis, LRTI, UTI, SSTI, abdominal infection; septicemia.

Dosage: IV

- Adults: Mild to moderate infection: 0.5–1 g every 8 hours
  Meningitis: 2 g every 8 hours
- Children > 3 months: Mild to moderate infection: 20 mg/kg 8 hours
  Meningitis: 40 mg/kg every 8 hours
- Neonates: 20 mg/kg/dose every 12 hours

Brands: 500 and 1000 mg Vial; Merogen, Meronem. 125, 250, 500 mg Vial; Ronem.

Nursing consideration: For IV use dilute in 10–20 ml of NS/D5W in a concentration of 50 mg/ml and infuse over 3–5 minutes. Prolonged use may cause superinfection. Use with caution in patients with history of seizures and CNS disease.

(C) ANTIBIOTICS—CEPHALOSPORINS

Includes: Four generations.

Action: Inhibits bacterial cell wall synthesis by binding to one or more of the penicillin binding proteins, resulting in cell death.

Side Effects: Common side effects are; N/V, diarrhea, rash. Serious are; seizures, serum sickness, pseudomembranous colitis, phlebitis.

General Nursing Considerations

- **Assess:** CBC, LFT, RFT, PT, culture and sensitivity; signs and symptoms of infection, history of previous reactions, signs and symptoms of anaphylaxis (rash, pruritus, wheezing, laryngeal edema). Assess NB for jaundice and hyperbilirubinemia if planning to use ceftriaxone. Presistent temperature elevation may be drug induced fever
- **Administration:** PO ± food and give round the clock. Monitor IV line for phlebitis and change site every 2–3 days. Keep a gap of 1 hour between aminoglycosides and cephalosporins if using concurrently, flush line between medication if using same line or use separate lines. For IV use dilute 1 g of cephalosporin in at least 10 ml and infuse over 3–5 minutes. For IM use reconstitute the dose in 3–3.5 ml of NS/SWI to achieve a concentration of 200–300 mg/ml. Nystatin may be given for secondary infection
- **Advise:** Take exactly as directed. Use caliberated caps and droppers for liquid preparations. Report signs and symptoms of superinfection, fever and diarrhea. Prolonged use may cause superinfection. Avoid alcohol, it may cause disulfiram like reaction
- **Desired Outcome:** Resolution of signs and symptoms of infection, decrease incidence of infection when used for prophylaxis.

FIRST GENERATION CEPHALOSPORINS

Include: 1. Cefadroxil 2. Cefazolin 3. Cephalexin

1. Cefadroxil

Uses: Streptococcal pharyngitis/tonsillitis, SSTI caused by streptococci or staphylococci, UTI caused by *E. coli*, etc.

Dosage: PO

- Adults: 1-2 g/day in 2 divided doses
- Infants and Children: 30 mg/kg/day in 2 divided doses (Max: 2 g/day).

Brands: 125, 250, 500 mg Tab;125 and 250 mg/5 ml Syp; Bicef, Cefodrox, Odoxil.

2. Cefazolin

Uses: Treatment of gram positive infection causing SSTI, RTI, UTI, preoperative prophylaxis, bacterial endocarditis, prophylaxis for dental and upper respiratory procedures.

Dosage: IM, IV

- Adults: Usual doses, 0.5-2 g every 6-8 hours.
  UTI: 1 g every 12 hours.
  Preoperative prophylaxis: 1 g 30-60 minutes before surgery, then 0.5-1 g every 8 hours for 24 hours.
  Infective endocarditis prophylaxis: 1-1.5 g 30 minutes before procedure
- Infants and children: Usual dosage, 50-100 mg/kg/day divided every 8 hours. Infective endocarditis prophylaxis: 25 mg/kg 30 minutes prior to procedure (Max: 1 g).

Brands: 250, 500 and 1000 mg Vial; Cefdin, Ozalin, Reflin.

Nursing consideration: For IV use dilute is NS/D_5W/RL to a concentration of 100 mg/ml and infuse over 3-5 minutes.

3. Cephalexin

Uses: Treatment of RTI, SSTI, GUTI and OM.

Dosage: PO

- Adults: 250-500 mg every 6 hours.
- Children: 25-100 mg/kg/day divided every 6-8 hours.

Brands: 125, 250, 500 mg Tab; 125 and 250 mg/5 ml Syp; 100 mg/ml Drops; Cephadex, Phexin, Sporidex.

SECOND GENERATION CEPHALOSPORINS

Includes: 1. Cefaclor 2. Cefprozil 3. Cefuroxime

1. Cefaclor

Uses: Treatment of OM, sinusitis, RTI, SSTI, UTI.

Dosage: PO

- Adults: 250–500 mg every 8 hours.
- Children > 1 month: 20–40 mg/kg/day divided every 8–12 hours.

Brands: 125, 250, 375 mg Tab; 125 mg/5 ml Syp; 50 mg/ml Drops; Distaclor, Keflor.

Nursing consideration: Keep a gap of 2 hours between antacids and cefaclor.

2. Cefprozil

Uses: Treatment of RTI, SSTI, OM.

Dosage: PO

- Adults and Children > 12 years: 250–500 mg every 12 hours.
- Children > 6 months: 15–20 mg/kg/day divided every 12 hours.

Brands: 250 and 500 mg Tab; CEF, Orprozil.

3. Cefuroxime

Uses: Treatment of URTI, LRTI, OM, maxillary sinusitis, UTI, SSTI, septicemia.

Dosage:

- Adults and children > 12 years (PO): Usual dosage: 250–500 mg twice daily
  Uncomplicated UTI: 125–250 mg every 12 hours
  Uncomplicated gonorrhea: 1 g single dose
- Infant ≥ 3 months and children upto 12 years:
  AOM, sinusitis: 30 mg/kg/day divided every 12 hours.
  Pharyngitis, tonsillitis: 20 mg/kg/day divided every 8 hours.
- Adults (IM, IV): 750–1.5 g every 8 hours.
- Children (IM, IV): 75–150 mg/kg/day divided every 8 hours.

Brands: 125, 250, 500 mg Tab; 125 mg/5 ml Syp; 250, 750 and 1500 mg Vial; Altacef, Cepokem, Widecef.

Nursing Consideration: As tablets have a bitter taste it should be swallowed whole. High fat meal diet increases drug bioavailability. For IV use dilute in NS/D_5W in a concentration of 30 mg/ml and infuse over 15–30 minutes.

THIRD GENERATION CEPHALOSPORINS

Include:

1. Cefdinir
2. Cefixime
3. Cefoperazone
4. Cefotaxime
5. Ceftamet
6. Ceftazidime
7. Ceftizoxime
8. Cefpodoxime
9. Ceftriaxone

1. Cefdinir

Uses: Treatment of RTI, SSTI, OM.

Dosage: PO

- Adults and Children > 12 years: 300 mg twice daily for 5–10 days
- Infants ≥ 6 months and children upto 12 years: 14 mg/kg/day divided every 12 hours for 5–10 days.

Brands: 100,150 mg Tab; 300 mg Cap; 125 mg/5 ml Syp; Aldinir, Rtist, Zinir.

Nursing Consideration: Do not give within 2 hours of antacids or iron administration as these decreases absorption by 40–80% respectively. Stools may initially turn red in color.

2. Cefixime

Uses: Treatment of UTI, OM, RTI, gonorrhea, typhoid.

Dosage: PO

- Adults and children > 12 years or > 50 kg: Usual dosage 400 mg/day divided every 12 hours
  Gonorrhea: 400 mg single dose along with azithromycin 1 g single dose or doxycycline 100 mg twice daily for 7 days
- Children upto 12 years: Usual dosage: 8 mg/kg/day divided every 12 hours
  Acute UTI: 16 mg/kg/day divided every 12 hours for 13 days
  Typhoid: 15–20 mg/kg/day divided every 12 hours

Brands: 100, 200 mg Tab; 50 and 100 mg/5 ml Syp; Biotax-O, Extacef, Zifi, Hifen.

3. Cefoperazone

Uses: Treatment of RTI, SSTI, UTI, septicemia.

Dosage: IM, IV.

- Adults: 2–4 g/day divided every 12 hours
- Infants and Children: 100–150 mg/kg/day divided every 12 hours.

Brands: 250, 500 and 1000 mg Vial; Magnamycin, Myticef.

Nursing Consideration: Specially monitor PT time. Disulfiram like reaction may occur if taken with alcohol. For IV use dilute each 1 g in 3 mL of SWI/NS and this is further diluted in 20–40 mL of NS in a concentration of 25–50 mg/mL and infuse over 15–30 minutes.

4. Cefotaxime

Uses: Treatment of LRTI, SSTI, GUTI, abdominal, meningitis and gonococcal infection in female.

Dosage: IM, IV

- Adults and Children > 12 years: 1–2 g every 6–8 hours.
- Children < 12 years and infants:
  ≤ 50 kg: 100–200 mg/kg/day divided every 6–8 hours. Meningitis: 200 mg/kg/day divided every 6 hours.
  > 50 kg: Moderate to severe infection: 1–2 g every 6–8 hours.

Brands: 125, 250, 500 and 1000 mg Vial; C-Tax, Clofaron, Omnicef.

Nursing Consideration: IV doses are given diluted in 50–100 ml of D5W/RL/NS in a concentration of 20–60 mg/ml and infused over 20–30 minutes. Rapid infusion over less than 1 minute may cause arrhythmias.

5. Ceftamet

Uses: Treatment of URTI, LRTI, gonorrhea.

Dosage:
- Adults and children ≥ 12 years: 500 mg twice daily
- Children < 12 years: 10 mg/kg twice daily.

Brands: 250 and 500 mg Tab; Altamet, Ultipime-O.

6. Ceftazidime

Uses: Treatment of RTI, SSTI, UTI, abdominal infections, septicemia, meningitis.

Dosage: IM, IV.
- Adults: 1–2 g every 8–12 hours usual doses. UTI: 250–500 mg every 12 hours
- Infants > 1 month and children: Usual doses 100–150 mg/kg/day divided every 8 hours. Meningitis: 150 mg/kg/day divided every 8 hours.

Brands: 250, 500 and 1000 mg Vial; C-Zid, Fortum, Tazid.

Nursing Consideration: For IV use dilute in NS/RL/D_5W in a concentration of 40 mg/ml and infuse over 15–30 minutes.

7. Ceftizoxime

Uses: Treatment of RTI, UTI, SSTI, gonorrhea, *H. influenzae* and meningitis.

Dosage: IM, IV.
- Adults: Usual dosage: 1–2 g every 8–12 hours
  Life-threatening infection: 3–4 g every 8 hours
  Uncomplicated gonorrhea (IM): 1 g single dose
- Children > 6 months: 150–200 mg/kg/day divided every 6–8 hours

Brands: 250 and 1000 mg Vial; Cefizox, Eldcef.

Nursing Consideration: For IV use dilute in 100 ml of NS/RL/D_5W in a concentration of 20 mg/ml and infuse over 15–30 minutes.

8. Cefpodoxime

Uses: Pneumonia, uncomplicated gonorrhea, SSTI, AOM, pharyngitis, tonsillitis, uncomplicated UTI.

Dosage: PO
- Adults: 100–400 mg/dose every 12 hours. Uncomplicated gonorrhea: 200 mg as a single dose
- Infants > 6 months and children: 10 mg/kg/day divided every 12 hours (Max: 200 mg BD).

Brands: 100, 200 mg Tab; 50 and 100 mg/5 ml Syp; Cefoprox, Cepodem, Doxcef.

Nursing Consideration: Do not administer within 2 hours of antacids or H_2 antagonists as these decreases absorption.

9. Ceftriaxone

Uses: Treatment of LRTI, SSTI, abdominal, UTI, sepsis, meningitis, gonococcal and salmonellosis.

Dosage: IM, IV

- Adults: Usual dosage: 1–2 g every 12–24 hours
  Gonorrhea: 250 mg IM single dose
  Meningitis: 2 g every 12 hours
- Children: Usual dosage: 50–75 mg/kg/day divided every 12–24 hous
  Meningitis: 80–100 mg/kg/day divided every 12 hours
  Gonorrhea: 125 mg IM single dose
- Neonates: 50 mg/kg/day divided every 12 hours

Brands: 125, 250, 500 and 1000 mg Vial; C-Tri, Cefaxone, Cefazone, Taxone.

Nursing Consideration: For IV dilute in NS/D_5W in a concentration of 40 mg/ml and infuse over 10–30 minutes.

FOURTH GENERATION CEPHALOSPORINS

Includes: 1. Cefepime 2. Cefpirome

1. Cefepime

Uses: Treatment of LRTI, SSTI, UTI, cellulitis, septicemia.

Dosage: IV

- Adults: Usual dosage 1–2 g every 12 hours. UTI: 500 mg every 12 hours
- Children 2 months–16 years, < 40 kg: 50 mg/kg/dose every 12 hours

Brands: 250, 500 and 1000 mg. vial; Cepime, Maxicef, Novapime.

Nursing Consideration: For IV use dilute is NS/RL/D5W in a concentration of 40 mg/ml and infuse over 20–30 minutes.

2. Cefpirome

Uses: Treatment of RTI, UTI, SSTI, septicemia.

Dosage: Adults (IV): 1–2 g every 12 hours.

Brands: 250, 500, 1000 mg Vial; Bacirom, Forgen.

Nursing Consideration: For IV use dilute in NS and infuse over 20–30 minutes.

(D) ANTIBIOTICS—FLUOROQUINOLONES

Include: 1. Ciprofloxacin 2. Gatifloxacin 3. Gemifloxacin 4. Levofloxacin 5. Lomefloxacin 6. Moxifloxacin 7. Norfloxacin 8. Ofloxacin 9. Sparfloxacin

Action: Inhibits bacterial DNA synthesis by inhibiting DNA gyrase resulting in death of susceptible bacteria.

Side Effects: Common side effects are; nausea, vomiting, diarrhea, headache, dizziness, insomnia, increased liver enzymes. Serious are; seizures, pseudomembranous colitis, anaphylaxis, SJS, arrhythmias.

General Nursing Considerations

- **Assess:** CBC, LFT, RFT, Blood sugar, PT, culture and sensitivity; signs and symptoms of infection and anaphylaxis
- **Administration:** Use with caution in CNS disorders, seizures and renal impairment. Avoid use in <18 years age group unless strongly indicated. If receiving anticoagulants and theophyllines, monitor closely; it may cause bleeding or seizures
- **Advise:** Take exactly as directed and for full course of therapy even if feeling better. Medicines containing antacids, iron or zinc will decrease their absorption if given concurrently. Maintain fluid intake of 1.5-2 L/day. It may cause dizziness and drowsiness so avoid activities requiring mental alertness. Report signs and symptoms of superinfection, fever and diarrhea. Patient with uncorrected hypokalemia, myocardial ischemia and bradycardia should avoid quinolones. Report any new onset pain or inflammation of tendon or extremity; tendon rupture may occur
- **Desired Outcome:** Resolution of signs and symptoms of infection.

1. Ciprofloxacin

Uses: Treatment of RTI, UTI, SSTI, bone and joint, *Mycobacterium tuberculosis*, shigella and salmonella.

Dosage:

- Adults: Most infections (PO): 250–750 mg every 12 hours. (IV): 200–400 mg every 12 hours.
  Gonorrhea: 250 mg single dose
  Uncomplicated UTI (PO): 500 mg every 24 hours for 3 days
  (IV): 200 mg every 12 hours for 7–14 days
  Complicated UTI (PO): 1000 mg every 24 hours for 7–14 days
  (IV): 400 mg every 24 hours for 7–14 days
- Children (PO, IV): 20–30 mg/kg/day divided every 12 hours (Max. PO: 1.5 g/day and IV: 800 mg/day).

Brands: 100, 250, 500 and 750 mg Tab; 2 mg/ml infusion; Cifran, Ciplox, Ciprobid.

Nursing Consideration: For IV use dilute in NS/D_5W in a concentration of 2 mg/ml and infuse over 60 minutes. Antacids and sucralfate may decrease absorption upto 90% if used concurrently, keep a gap of 2–4 hours.

2. Gatifloxacin

Uses: Treatment of UTI, RTI, gonorrhea.

Dosage:

- Adults (PO, IV): 400 mg once daily. Give for 3 days in UTI and single dose in gonorrhea
- Children (PO): 10 mg/kg/day single dose.

Brands: 200 and 400 mg Tab; 2 mg/ml infusion; Gaity, Gatilox, Gator.

3. Gemifloxacin

Uses: Acute bacterial exacerbation of chronic bronchitis, CAP.

Dosage: PO ± food.

- Adults: Chronic bronchitis: 320 mg single dose for 5 days.
  CAP: 320 mg single dose for 5–7 days.

Brands: 320 mg Tab; Floxigem, Gemif, Zemi.

Nursing consideration: Should be given 2 hours before or after antacids or other products containing calcium, magnesium, aluminium, iron, zinc.

4. Levofloxacin

Uses: Treatment of LRTI, maxillary sinusitis, SSTI, nosocomial infection, UTI, chronic bacterial prostatitis.

Dosage: PO, IV.

- Adults: 250–750 mg/day once daily
- Children: 5–10 mg/kg/day once daily (Max: 500 mg).

Brands: 250, 500, 750 mg Tab; 5 mg/ml infusion; Fynal, Lee, Levobact.

Nursing Consideration: PO ± food. IV doses given diluted in NS/D5W in a concentration of 5 mg/ml and infuse over 60–90 minutes. Rapid infusion may cause hypotension. Administer PO 2 hours after antacids.

5. Lomefloxacin

Uses: Treatment of UTI and surgical prophylaxis.

Dosage: PO ± food.

Adults: UTI: 400 mg once daily for 10–14 days

Surgical prophylaxis: 400 mg once daily 1–6 hours before procedure.

Brands: 400 mg Tab; Floxaday, Lomedon, Lomitas.

6. Moxifloxacin

Uses: Treatment of CAP, acute bacterial exacerbation of chronic bronchitis, SSTI, sinusitis, abdomen infection.

Dosage: Adults (PO, IV): 400 mg once daily (CAP: 7–14 days, chronic bronchitis: 5 days, SSTI: 7–21 days, sinusitis: 10 days).

Brands: 400 mg Tab; 4 mg/ml Inj; Moxif, Staxom.

Nursing Consideration: PO + food. Should be taken 4 hours before or after antacids or product containing iron, zinc, calcium, aluminium, magnesium. IV dose should be given over 60 minutes.

7. Norfloxacin

Uses: Treatment of UTI, prostatitis, gonorrhea, gastroenteritis.

Dosage:

- Adults (PO): 400 mg once daily (UTI: 10–15 days, prostatitis: 4–6 weeks, gastroenteritis: 3–5 days, gonorrhea: 800 mg single dose)
- Children (PO): 6–12 mg/kg/day divided every 12 hours.

Brands: 200, 400 mg Tab; Norflox, Quinobid, Norbactin.

Nursing Consideration: PO 1 hour before or 2 hours after meals.

8. Ofloxacin

Uses: Treatment of CAP, UTI, typhoid, prostatitis, PID, gonorrhea.

Dosage: PO, IV.

- Adults: Most infection 200–400 mg every 12 hours
  Gonorrhea: 400 mg single dose
  UTI: 200 mg every 12 hourly for 7–10 days
  CAP: 400 mg every 12 hourly for 10 days
  Typhoid: 200–400 mg every 12 hourly for 7–14 days
  Prostatitis: 300 mg every 12 hourly for 6 weeks
- Children (PO): 15 mg/kg/day divided every 12 hourly
  (IV): 5–10 mg/kg/day divided every 12 hourly.

Brands: 200, 400 mg Tab; 2 mg/ml infusion; 50 mg/5 ml Syp; OF, Zenflox, ZO.

Nursing Consideration: PO given 1 hour before or 2 hours after meal. IV doses given slowly over 30 minutes.

9. Sparfloxacin

Uses: Treatment of CAP, acute bacterial exacerbation of chronic bronchitis.

Dosage: Adults (PO): 100–300 mg/day in single or divided doses.

Brands: 100, 200 mg Tab; Flospar, Sparbact, Zospar.

(E) ANTIBIOTICS—IMIDAZOLES

Include: 1. Metronidazole 2. Ornidazole 3. Tinidazole

Action: Metronidazole disrupts bacterial DNA and protein synthesis. Tinidazole causes release of free nitroradicals which has antiprotozoal activity.

Side Effects: Nausea, vomiting, metallic taste, dry mouth, headache, dizziness, transient leukopenia, disulfiram like reaction with alcohol, peripheral neuropathy.

General Nursing Considerations

- **Assess:** CBC, LFT, culture and sensitivity; input and output; signs and symptoms of infection; neurological status
- **Advise:** Take exactly as directed for full course. Avoid alcohol. Frequent mouth rinses, good oral hygiene, chewing gum may decrease dry mouth sensation. Partners of trichomoniasis patient should be treated concurrently and use condom to prevent reinfection
- **Desired Outcome:** Resolution of infection.

1. Metronidazole

Uses: Treatment of anaerobic infection: Intra-abdominal, SSTI, LRTI, CNS, gynecologic, septicemia; amebic dysentery, amebic liver abscess, trichomoniasis, giardiasis.

Dosage: PO + food.

- Adults: Anaerobic infection (PO, IV): 30 mg/kg/day divided every 6 hours
  Amebiasis (PO): 500–750 mg every 8 hours
  Other parasites (PO): 250 mg every 8 hours
- Children: Anaerobic infection (PO, IV): 30 mg/kg/day divided every 6 hours
  Amebiasis (PO): 35–50 mg/kg/day divided every 8 hours
  Other parasites (PO): 15–30 mg/kg/day divided every 8 hours

Brands: 200 and 400 mg Tab; 200 mg/5 ml Syp; 5 mg/ml infusion; Aldezole, Metrogyl.

Nursing Consideration: PO ± food. IV given slowly over 30–60 minutes in a concentration of 5–8 mg/ml. Use with caution in patient with edema or those on corticosteroid therapy. With IV therapy assess for sodium retention.

2. Ornidazole

Uses: Treatment of amebiasis, giardiasis, trichomoniasis, amebic liver abscess, anaerobic bacterial infection.

Dosage: PO + food.

- Adults: Amebiasis (PO): 0.5 g/dose every 12 hours for 5–10 days
  Other infection (IV): 0.5–1 gm/dose every 12 hours for 5–7 days
- Children: Amebiasis (PO): 40 mg/kg/day divided every 12 hours for 5–10 day
  Other infection (IV): 20–30 mg/kg every 12 hours for 5–10 days.

Brands: 500 mg Tab; 5 mg/ml infusion; Dazolic, Ornida.

3. Tinidazole

Uses: Treatment of amebiasis, giardiasis, trichomoniasis.

Dosage: PO

- Adults: 2 g/dose. Single dose for giardiasis and trichomoniasis and 3–5 days for amebic infection
- Children: 50 mg/kg/day. Single dose for giardiasis and 3–5 days for amebic infection.

Brands: 300, 500 and 1000 mg Tab; Tina, Tiniba.

(F) ANTIBIOTICS—MACROLIDES

Include:

1. Azithromycin
2. Clarithromycin
3. Erythromycin
4. Roxithromycin

Action: Inhibits bacterial RNA dependent protein synthesis by binding to the 50s ribosomal subunit.

Side Effects: Nausea, vomiting, abdominal pain, increased liver enzymes, cholestatic jaundice, headache, dizziness, rash, pruritus, anaphylaxis, metallic taste, pseudomembranous colitis.

General Nursing Considerations

- **Assess:** CBC, LFT, RFT, blood sugar, culture and sensitivity; assess for signs and symptoms of infection and anaphylaxis
- **Administration:** Use caliberated cups and dropper for liquid preparations
- **Advise:** Take exactly as directed and for full course of therapy even if feeling well. Report signs and symptoms of superinfection, fever and diarrhea, may cause dizziness and drowsiness so avoid activities requiring mental alertness
- **Desired Outcome:** Resolution of signs and symptoms of infection; endocarditis prophylaxis as applicable to particular drug.

1. Azithromycin

Uses: Treatment of URTI, LRTI, CAP, SSTI, AOM, Urethritis and cervicitis.

Dosage: PO, should be given 1 hour before or 2 hours after meals.

- Adults and children >16 years: RTI, SSTI: 500 mg on day 1, then 250 mg/day once daily for 5 days
  Nongonococcal urethritis and cervicitis: 1 g single dose
  Gonococcal infection: 2 g single dose
  Endocarditis prophylaxis: 500 mg 1 hour before procedure
- Children > 6 months:
  Pharyngitis/tonsillitis: 12 mg/kg/day once daily for 5 days
  Endocarditis prophylaxis: 15 mg/kg/dose 1 hour before procedure.

Brands: 100, 250, 500 mg Tab; 100 and 200 mg/5 ml Syp; Azec, Azest, Azithral.

Nursing Consideration: Avoid Al or Mg containing antacids simultaneously.

2. Clarithromycin

Uses: Treatment of URTI, LRTI, AOM, SSTI, endocarditis prophylaxis.

Dosage: PO + food.

- Adults: Most of the infection: 250 mg every 12 hours for 7–14 days
  Endocarditis prophylaxis: 500 mg 1 hour before procedure
- Children: Most of the infection: 15 mg/kg/day divided every 12 hours for 7–14 days
  Endocarditis prophylaxis: 15 mg/kg 1 hour before procedure.

Brands: 125, 250, 500 mg Tab; 125 mg/5 ml Syp; Clarie, Claribid, Maclar.

3. Erythromycin

Uses: Treatment of URTI, LRTI, pharyngitis, SSTI, diphtheria, pertussis.

Dosage: PO + food.

- Adults: 250 mg every 6 hours or 500 mg every 12 hours.
- Children: 30–50 mg/kg/day divided every 6–8 hours (Max: 1 g/day).

Brands: 125, 250, 500 mg Tab; Althrocin, Erycin. 125 mg/5 ml Syp; Althrocin, Eltocin, Eromed.

4. Roxithromycin

Uses: Treatment of URTI, LRTI, syphilis, gonorrhea.

Dosage: PO ± food.

- Adults: 150–300 mg twice daily
- Children: 5–8 mg/kg/day divided every 12 hours for 7 days

Brands: 50, 150 mg Tab; 50 mg/5 ml Syp; Biorox, Roxid, Roxyrol.

(G) ANTIBIOTICS—PENICILLINS

Includes: 1. Amoxicillin 2. Amoxicillin + Clavulanic acid 3. Ampicillin 4. Ampicillin + Sulbactum 5. Benzathine penicillin-G 6. Penicillin-G 7. Penicillin-V 8. Piperacillin + Tazobactum 9. Procaine penicillin-G 10. Ticarcillin + Clavulanic acid

Action: Binds to one or more of the penicillin binding proteins during multiplication causing cell death.

Side Effects: Common side effects are; nausea, vomiting, diarrhea, raised liver enzymes, rashes, superinfection, phlebitis. Serious are; seizures, anaphylaxis, pseudomembranous colitis. Ticarcillin in addition may also cause hypokalemia, CHF, hypernatremia.

General Nursing Considerations

- **Assess:** CBC, LFT, RFT, serum electrolytes; BT, PT; Vitals; culture and sensitivity; previous history of allergic reaction; signs and symptoms of infection and anaphylaxis. Patients with history of asthma, hay fever, urticaria are more prone to allergic reactions
- **Administration:** Use caliberated dropper and caps for liquid preparations. Change IV site every 2–3 days. For IM use reconstitute in D_5W/NS and shake well before injection, give at a slow consistent rate to prevent blockage of needle. If penicillin and aminoglycosides are used concurrently, give from separate site and keep a gap of 1 hour between them. Keep epinephrine, antihistamine and resuscitation equipment ready to manage anaphylaxis. Keep ambulatory patient under observation for 30 minutes to assess for anaphylaxis. Do not rub long-acting penicillin products after injection
- **Advise:** Take exactly as directed even if feeling well. Report signs and symptoms of super-infection, allergy, diarrhea, bloody stools, fever. Take PO with a glass of water 1 hour before or 2 hours after meal
- **Desired Outcome:** Resolution of signs and symptoms of infection.

1. Amoxicillin

Uses: Treatment of RTI, SSTI, OM, sinusitis, GUTI, endocarditis prophylaxis.

Dosage: PO ± meals.

- Adults: Most infections: 250–500 mg every 8 hours. Endocarditis prophylaxis: 1 hour before procedure

- Children: Most infection: 25–50 mg/kg/day divided every 8 hours. Endocarditis prophylaxis: 50 mg/kg 1 hour before procedure.

Brands: 125, 250 mg Tab; 250, 500 mg Cap; 125 mg/5 ml Syp; Aristomox, Mox, Novamox.

Nursing Consideration: May cause tooth discoloration specially in younger patients.

2. Amoxicillin+Clavulanic acid

Clavulanic acid binds to beta lactamase enzyme capable of inactivating amoxicillin.

Uses: Treatment of RTI, SSTI, OM, sinusitis, UTI.

Dosage: Based on amoxicillin component. Give IV/PO. PO should be given at the beginning of meals and should not be given with high fat diet.

- Adults and children ≥ 40 kg: Mild infection; 250 mg every 8 hours. Severe infection and RTI; 500 mg every 8 hours
- Children < 40 kg: 20–45 mg/kg/day divided every 8 hours.

Brands: Amoxicillin+Clavulanic acid: 250 + 125 and 500 + 125 mg Tab; 200 + 28.5 mg Syp; Clavam, Bestomox, Hibrid. 250 + 50, 500 + 100, 1000 + 200 mg Inj; Clavam, Augmentin.

3. Ampicillin

Uses: Treatment of RTI, SSTI, OM, sinusitis, GUTI, septicemia, endocarditis prophylaxis, meningitis.

Dosage:

- Adults: Most infections (PO): 250–500 mg every 6 hours (IM, IV): 500 mg–3 g every 6 hours. Endocarditis prophylaxis: 2 g, 30 minutes before procedure
- Children: Most infections (PO): 50–100 mg/kg/day divided every 6 hours (IM, IV): 100–200 mg/kg/day divided every 6 hours.
  Meningitis (IM, IV): 200–400 mg/kg/day divided every 6 hours.
  Endocarditis prophylaxis: 50 mg/kg, 30 minutes before procedure.

Brands: 125, 250 mg Tab; 250, 500 mg Cap; 125 and 250 mg/5 ml Syp; Ampilin, Aristocillin, Roscilin.

Nursing Consideration: PO given 1 hour before or 2 hours after meals. For IV use dilute in SWI in a concentration of 30–100 mg/mL and infuse at the rate of 100 mg/min. Use solution within 1 hour of reconstitution.

4. Ampicillin+Sulbactum

Uses: Treatment of RTI, SSTI, OM, sinusitis, GUTI, septicemia, meningitis.

Dosage: IM, IV. Based on ampicillin component.

- Adults: 1–2 g every 6–8 hours
- Children: 100–200 mg/kg/day divided every 6 hours. Meningitis: 200–400 mg/kg/day divided every 6 hours.

Brands: Ampicillin+Sulbactum: 1 g+0.5 g Inj; Ampitum, Betamp.

Nursing Consideration: For IV use dilute in SWI in a concentration of 50 mg/mL and infuse over 15–20 minutes.

5. Benzathine Penicillin-G

Uses: Treatment of Streptococcal pharyngitis, syphilis, rheumatic fever prophylaxis.

Dosage: IM

- Streptococcal URTI: Adults: 1.2 million units single dose
  Children: < 27 kg: 300,000–600,000 units single dose
  ≥ 27 kg: 900,000 units single dose
- Rheumatic fever prophylaxis: Adults: 1.2 million units every 3–4 weeks
  Children: 25,000–50,000 units/kg every 3–4 weeks.

Brands: 6, 12 and 24 lakh unit vials; Pencom LA, Penidura LA.

6. Penicillin-G/Crystalline Penicillin

Uses: Treatment of pneumonia, septicemia, meningitis, endocarditis.

Dosage: IM, IV.

- Adults: 2–24 million units/day divided every 4–6 hours
- Children: Most infection: 100,000–250,000 units/kg/day divided every 4–6 hours. Severe infection: 250,000–400,000 units/kg/day divided every 4–6 hours.

Brands: 5,10 lac units; Benzyl penicillin.

Nursing Consideration: Large doses of Penicillin-G potassium may cause hyperkalemia. When using penicillin-G sodium in large doses always monitor serum sodium levels in patient with HT and CHF. For IV use dilute in NS/SWI in a concentration of 50,000–100,000 units/mL and infuse over 15–30 minutes.

7. Penicillin-V Potassium

Uses: Mild to moderate RTI, UTI; Prophylaxis of pneumococcal infection and rheumatic fever.

Dosage: PO ± food.

- Adults and Children ≥ 12 years: Most infections: 250–500 mg every 6–8 hours
- Children <12 years: Most infections: 25–50 mg/kg/day divided every 6–8 hours
- Rheumatic fever prophylaxis: 125–250 mg every 12 hours.

Brands: 125, 250 mg Tab; Kaypen.

8. Piperacillin+Tazobactum

Uses: Treatment of sepsis, LRTI, UTI, SSTI, CAP, abdominal, gynecological infections.

Dosage: IV. Dosage is based on piperacillin component.

- Adults: 3–4.5 g every 6 hours
- Infants and children: 100–300 mg/kg/day divided every 6–8 hours.

Brands: Piperacillin+Tazobactum: 2+0.25 and 4+0.5 g Vial; Cidal, Pipzo, Tazotum.

Nursing Consideration: Dilute each 1 g of piperacillin in 5 mL of NS/D5W/SWI and this is further diluted in 50–100 mL and infused over 30 minutes.

9. Procaine Penicillin-G/Aquaous Penicillin

Uses: Treatment of RTI, SSTI, *T pallidum* and other susceptible infections.

Dosage: IM

- Adults: 600,000–1.2 million units/day as a single dose
- Children: 25,000–50,000 units/kg/day divided every 12 hours.

Brands: 4 and 10 lac units Vial; Sodicillin.

10. Ticarcillin + Clavulanic acid

Uses: Treatment of LRTI, SSTI, UTI, septicemia, abdominal and gynecological infection.

Dosage: IV. Dosage based on Ticarcillin component.

- Adults and children >16 years: 3 g every 4–6 hours
- Children 3 months–16 years: 200–300 mg/kg/day divided every 4–6 hours.

Brands: 3.1 g vials; Timentin

Nursing Consideration: For IV use dilute in NS/SWI to achieve a concentration of 200 mg/mL, dilute it further to achieve a concentration of 10–100 mg/mL and infuse over 30 minutes.

(H) ANTIBIOTICS—TETRACYCLINES

Includes: 1. Doxycycline 2. Minocycline 3. Tetracycline

Action: Inhibits protein synthesis by binding to 30s ribosomal subunits of bacteria.

Side Effects: Common side effects are; nausea, vomiting, diarrhea, esophagitis, hepatotoxicity, rashes, photosensitivity, dizziness, raised ICP, discoloration of nails and teeth, candidiasis.

General Nursing Considerations

- **Assess:** CBC, RFT, LFT, input and output; culture and sensitivity; bowel pattern; signs and symptoms of infection. Observe for signs and symptoms of enterocolitis (diarrhea, fever, abdominal pain, scanty urine) for these drug may need to stopped.
- **Administration:** PO 1 hour before or 2 hours after meals. It should not be used in < 8 years of age. It may cause retardation in skeletal development, softening of bones and teeth if used in < 8 years of age and during second half of pregnancy
- **Advise:** Take exactly as directed even if feeling better. Minocycline may cause dizziness and drowsiness, so avoid activities requiring mental alertness. Avoid exposure to sunlight and artificial light. Do not take milk and milk products along with tetracycline. Avoid antacids, iron, zinc, calcium, aluminium containing drugs within 2–3 hours of tetracyclines. Report signs and symptoms of superinfection. They may cause anal itching which can be prevented by cleansing anal area with water after each bowel movement
- **Desired Outcome:** Decrease in signs and symptoms of infection.

1. Doxycycline

Uses: Treatment of GUTI, RTI, PID, gonorrhea, malaria prophylaxis.

Dosage: PO

- Adults and children >8 years and >45 kg:
  Most of the infections: 50–100 mg every 12 hours
  Gonorrhea: 100 mg 12 hours for 7 days
  Malaria prophylaxis: 100 mg once daily, starting 2 days before journey
- Children >8 years ≤45 kg: 2–4 mg/kg/day divided every 12 hours.

Brands: 100 mg Tab and Cap; Microdox, Tetradox. 50, 100 and 200 mg Cap; Doxy-1.

2. Minocycline

Uses: Treatment of PID, STD, acne, nongonococcal urethritis and cervicitis.

Dosage: PO

- Adults: 100–200 mg initially then 100 mg every 12 hours
- Children ≥8 years: Initially 4 mg/kg, then 2 mg/kg every 12 hours.

Brands: 50, 100 mg Tab; Minolox. 50, 100 mg Cap; Cynomycin.

3. Tetracycline

Uses: Treatment of cholera, acne, CAP, STD.

Dosage: PO

- Adults: 250–500 mg/dose every 6–12 hours
- Children >8 years: 25–50 mg/kg/day divided every 6 hours.

Brands: 500 mg Tab; Hostacycline, Tetrabact. 250, 500 mg Cap; Achromycin, Tetlis.

(I) ANTIBIOTICS—MISCELLANEOUS

1. Aztreonam

Uses: Treatment of LRTI, SSTI, GUTI, septicemia, abdominal infection.

Dosage: IM, IV.

- Adults: 500 mg–1 g every 8–12 hours
- Children >1 month: 90–120 mg/kg/day divided every 6–8 hours.

Brands: 0.5, 1, 2 g Inj; Azenam, Aztreo, Trezam.

Side Effects: Common side effects are; nausea, vomiting, diarrhea, pseudomembranous colitis, rash, phlebitis, raised liver enzymes. Serious side effects being; hypotension, seizures, anaphylaxis.

Nursing Consideration: For IV use dilute in NS to achieve a concentration of 20 mg/mL and infuse over 20–60 minutes.

2. Chloramphenicol

Uses: Treatment of bacterial meningitis, brain abscess, *H. influenzae* infection, salmonella, etc.

Dosage: PO, 1 hour before or 2 hours after meals.

- Adults: 50 mg/kg/day divided every 6 hours
- Infants and children: 50–75 mg/kg/day divided every 6 hours.

Brands: 250 and 500 mg Cap; 125 mg/5 ml Syp; Aglomycetin, Fencol, Paraxin.

Side Effects: Common side effects are; nausea, vomiting, diarrhea, headache, peripheral neuropathy, optic neuritis. Serious side effects are; aplastic anemia, bone marrow suppression, gray baby syndrome.

Nursing Consideration: Monitor CBC. Its use may decrease intestinal absorption of Vitamin B_{12}. Avoid alcohol, NSAIDs and salicylates.

3. Clindamycin

Uses: Treatment of SSTI, RTI, septicemia, abdominal, gynecological infections; endocarditis prophylaxis.

Dosage:

- Adults (PO): 150–450 mg/dose every 6–8 hours
  (IM, IV): 1.2–1.8 g/day divided every 6–12 hours
- Children (PO): 10–30 mg/kg/day divided every 6–8 hours
  (IM, IV): 25–40 mg/kg/day divided every 6–8 hours.

Brands: 150, 300 mg Cap; 150 mg/ml Syp; 150 mg/ml Inj; Clincin, Dalcinex.

Side Effects: Nausea, vomiting, headache, dizziness, phlebitis, pseudomembranous colitis.

Nursing Consideration: Monitor CBC, RFT, LFT, culture and sensitivity; signs and symptoms of infection and superinfection. PO ± food. Maximum dose permitted via IM route is 600 mg. For IV use dilute in NS/RL/D5W to achieve a concentration of 18 mg/mL and infuse at the maximum rate of 30 mg/min. Rapid IVP may cause hypotension and CR arrest.

4. Lincomycin

Uses: Treatment of serious anaerobic infection.

Dosage:

- Adults (PO): 500 mg/dose every 6–8 hours
  (IM): 600 mg/dose 1–2 times/day. (IV): 0.6–1 g 2–3 times/day
- Children >1 month (PO): 30–60 mg/kg/day divided every 8–12 hours.
  (IM, IV): 10–20 mg/kg/day divided every 12 hours.

Brands: 200, 500 mg Cap; 125 mg/5 mL Syp; 300 mg/mL Inj; Lincozin, Lynx.

Side Effects: Refer clindamycin.

5. Linezolid

Uses: Treatment of complicated SSTI; hospital and community acquired pneumonia.

Dosage: PO, IV

- Adults: 400-600 mg every 12 hours
- Infants and children: 10 mg/kg/dose every 8 hours.

Brands: 600 mg Tab; 2 mg/mL infusion; Linospan, Linox, Lizolid.

Side Effects: Common side effects are; nausea, vomiting, diarrhea, headache. Serious side effects are; pseudomembranous colitis, thrombocytopenia, optic and peripheral neuropathy.

Nursing Consideration: PO±food. Monitor CBC, platelet count; acidosis. For IV use dilute in NS/RL in a concentration of 2 mg/mL and infuse over 30–120 minutes.

6. Nitazoxanide

Uses: Treatment of diarrhea caused by amebiasis, giardiasis, *C. parvum.*

Dosage: PO+food.

- Adults and children >12 years: 500 mg every 12 hours for 3 days
- Children: 4–11 years; 200 mg every 12 hours for 3 days. 1 to <4 years; 100 mg every 12 hours for 3 days.

Brands: 200, 500 mg Tab; 100 mg/5 mL Syp; Nizonide, Zoxakind.

Side Effects: Abdominal pain, diarrhea, vomiting, headache, yellow discoloration of eyes and urine, diaphoresis, pruritus.

7. Nitrofurantoin

Uses: Treatment and Prevention of UTI.

Dosage: PO + food.

UTI: Treatment: Adults: 50–100 mg every 6–8 hours. Children: 5–7 mg/kg/day divided every 6 hours.

UTI: Prophylaxis: Adults: 50–100 mg single evening dose. Children: 1–2 mg/kg/day single evening dose.

Brands: 50 and 100 mg Tab; Furadantin.

Side Effects: Common side effects being; anorexia, nausea, vomiting, drowsiness, brown discoloration of urine. Serious side effects include; hemolytic anemia, anaphylaxis, pseudomembranous colitis.

Nursing Consideration: Assess for signs and symptoms of UTI; input and output; CBC. It should not be used to treat UTI in febrile infants and young children with renal involvement.

8. Trimethoprim+Sulfamethoxazole.

Uses: Treatment of UTI, typhoid, Shigella enteritis, AOM, Pneumocystis carinii pneumonia.

Dosage: PO on empty stomach.

Adults and children >2 months; Mild to moderate infection: 6–12 mg of TMP/kg/day divided every 12 hours

Serious infection: 15–20 mg of TMP/kg/day divided every 12 hours.

Brands: TMP+SMX: 80+400 and 20+100 mg Tab; 40+200 mg/5 mL Syp; Bactrim, Ciplin, Septran.

Side Effects: Common side effects being; nausea, vomiting, diarrhea, cholestatic jaundice, rashes, headache. Serious effects include; erythema multiforme, SJS, pseudomembranous colitis, hepatic necrosis, megaloblastic anemia.

9. Vancomycin

Uses: (IV): Pneumonia, meningitis, endocarditis, septicemia, osteomyelitis.

(PO): Staphylococcal enterocolitis, antibiotic associated colitis.

Dosage:

- Severe infection (IV): Adults: 500 mg every 6 hours or 1 g every 12 hours
  Children: 40–60 mg/kg/day divided every 6–8 hours
- Colitis (PO): Adults: 125–500 mg every 6 hours
  Children: 40 mg/kg/day divided every 6 hours for 7–10 days.

Brands: 250 mg Cap; Vanlid. 500 and 1000 mg Vial; Vancomycin-CP, Vansafe.

Side Effects: Nausea, vomitting, ototoxicity, phlebitis, nephrotoxicity, fever, low back pain.

Nursing Consideration:

- **Assess:** BP, pulse; CBC, urine, RFT, culture sensitivity; input and output, weight; signs and symptoms of superinfection and infection
- **Administration:** Dilute 500 mg in 10 mL of SWI which is further diluted in 100 mL NS/RL to achieve a concentration of 5 mg/mL and this is then infused over 60 minutes. Rapid intfusion may cause red man syndrome. It may cause maculopapular rash over face, neck, trunk and upper extremity, therefore to prevent it slow the infusion rate and antihistamines administration just before infusion may also prevent it
- **Advise:** Report signs and symptoms of tinnitus, vertigo, hearing problem and allergy.

Chapter

8 Anticholinergics

Includes: 1. Atropine 2. Dicyclomine 3. Diphenoxylate 4. Glycopyrrolate 5. Hyoscyamine 6. Ipratropium 7. Oxybutynin 8. Propantheline 9. Tolterodine 10. Trihexyphenidyl

Action: Inhibits the action of acetylcholine at receptor sites.

Side Effects: Common side effects being; dry mouth, constipation, drowsiness, dizziness, nausea, blurred vision, dry eyes, disturbed urinary voiding pattern, tachycardia, decreased sweating.

General Nursing Considerations

- **Assess:** HR, BP, ECG, input and output, chest pain, abdominal distension, bowel sounds, stool pattern, urine voiding pattern, respiration. Asthma, glaucoma or duodenal ulcers are contraindication for anticholinergic therapy
- **Administration:** Give parenteral doses with patient in supine position to avoid postural hypotension
- **Advise:** It should be taken exactly as advised. Maintain good oral hygiene, frequent oral rinses to decrease dry mouth. Increase fluid, bulk, exercise to prevent constipation. Change position slowly to avoid orthostatic hypotension. Avoid activities requiring alertness. Some drugs impair heat regulation, so hot environment and extremes of temperature should be avoided. Dry mouth and blurred vision, have to be tolerated. Night vision may be impaired.

1. Atropine

Uses: Preoperative medication to decrease salivation and secretions, sinus bradycardia, reversal of the muscarinic effect of cholinergic agents (neostigmine, pyridostigmine), antidote for organophosphate or carbamate poisoning, exercise induced bronchospasm.

Dosage:

- Preanesthetic: IM, IV, SC

  Adults: 0.4–0.6 mg, 30–60 minutes preoperatively

Children >5 kg: 0.01–0.02 mg/kg/dose 30–60 minutes preoperatively
Children <5 kg: 0.02 mg/kg/dose 30–60 minutes preoperatively

- Bradycardia:
  Adults (IV): 0.5–1 mg every 5 minutes (max. total dose is 2 mg)
  Children (IV, IT): 0.02 mg/kg (min. dose is 0.1 mg and max is 0.5 mg)
- Reversal of muscarinic effects:
  Adults (IV): 0.6–12 mg for each 0.5–2.5 mg of neostigmine or 10–20 mg of pyridostigmine
- Organophosphate and carbamate poisoning:
  Adults (IV): 1–2 mg/dose every 10–20 minutes until dry flushed skin, tachycardia, fever seen then every 1–4 hourly for at least 24 hours
  Children (IV): 0.02–0.05 mg/kg every 10–20 minutes until atropine effects seen then every 1–4 hourly for at least 24 hours
- Bronchospasm (Inhalation):
  Adults: 0.025–0.05 mg/kg/dose every 4–6 hours as needed (Max: 2.5 mg/dose)
  Children: 0.03–0.05 mg/kg/dose every 4–6 hours as needed (Max: 2.5 mg/dose).

Brands: 0.6 mg/mL Inj; Tropine, ATP.

Nursing Consideration: IV should be given undiluted by rapid IV injection as slow push may result in paradoxical bradycardia. For intratracheal use, dilute in 3–5 ml of Normal Saline (NS) followed by several PPV. Harmless flushing of face and trunk may occur 15–20 minutes after IM administration.

Desired outcome: Increase in HR, decrease in secretions and reversal of muscarinic effects.

2. Dicyclomine

Uses: Treatment of functional disturbances of GI motility (IBS, GI spasm, diarrhea, peptic ulcer).

Dosage:

- Adults (PO): 10–20 mg 3–4 times/day. (IM): 20 mg every 6 hours as needed
- Children ≥ 12 years (PO): 10 mg 3–4 times/day
- Children 6 months—2 years (PO): 5–10 mg 3–4 times/day.

Brands: 20 mg Tab; Coligon. 10 mg/mL Inj; Clomin, Centwin.

Nursing Consideration: Assess for symptoms of IBS (abdominal cramps, mucus in stool, alternating diarrhea and constipation). Children with Down's syndrome, spastic paralysis or brain damage are more sensitive to toxic effects.

3. Diphenoxylate

For details refer—Antidiarrheals (Chapter 13).

4. Glycopyrrolate

Uses: Given preoperatively to decrease salivation and excessive respiratory secretions. It is used as an adjunct in the treatment of peptic ulcer disease. Also used for reversal of neuromuscular blockage.

Dosage:

- Preanesthetic: Given 30–60 minutes before procedure
  Adults (IM): 4.4 µg/kg
  Children (IM): <2 years, 4.4–8.8 µg/kg; >2 years, 4.4 µg/kg
- Peptic ulcer (IM, IV):
  Adults: 0.1–0.2 mg, 3–4 times/day
- Cholinergic adjunct (IV):
  Adults and children: 200 µg for each 1 mg of neostigmine or 5 mg of pyridostigmine.

Brands: 0.2 mg/mL Inj; Glypyrolate, Vagolate.

Nursing Consideration: IM doses can be given undiluted. IV doses can be given diluted in RL/NS/D5W in a 2 µg/mL dilution over 15–20 minutes. Desired outcome is decrease in secretion, motility and pain in peptic ulcer disease and reversal of cholinergic effects.

5. Hyoscyamine

Uses: Treatment of GI tract disorders caused by spasm, peptic ulcer, hypermotility disorders of lower urinary tract, infant colic.

Dosage:

- GI tract disorders:
  Adults and Children >12 years (IM, IV): 0.25–0.5 mg at 4 hours interval for 1–4 doses. (PO): 0.125–0.25 mg every 4 hours as needed
  Children: 2–12 years (PO): 0.0625–0.125 mg every 4 hours as needed
- Hypermotility of lower urinary tract:
  Adults (PO): 0.15–0.3 mg, 4 times/day.

Brands: 10 mg Tab; 7.5 mg/5 mL Syp; 20 mg/mL Inj; Buscopan.

Nursing Consideration: Give PO before meals. IV doses given diluted in 10 mL of sterile water.

6. Ipratropium

For details refer—antiasthmatics (Chapter 6).

7. Oxybutynin

Uses: Relief of urinary symptoms associated with neurogenic bladder and overactive bladder.

Dosage: PO±food.

- Adults: 2.5–5 mg, 2 or 3 times/day
- Children >5 years: 2.5 mg, 2 or 3 times/day.

Brands: 2.5 and 5 mg Tab; Cystran, Oxyspas.

Nursing Consideration: Relief of frequency, urgency, nocturia and incontinence.

8. Propantheline

Uses: As an adjunct in peptic ulcer, IBS, urinary bladder and ureteral spasm.

Dosage: PO

- Adults: 15 mg, 3 times/day, before meals and 30 mg at bed time
- Children: 1-2 mg/kg/day in 3-4 divided doses.

Brands: 15 mg Tab; Probanthine, Spastheline.

9. Tolterodine

Uses: Treatment of symptoms caused by overactive bladder.

Dosage: PO±food.

Adults: 2 mg BD.

Brands: 1 and 2 mg Tab; Terol, Tolter.

Nursing Consideration: Decrease in frequency and urge incontinence.

10. Trihexyphenidyl

For details refer—antiparkinson agents (Chapter 21).

Chapter 9 Anticoagulants

Includes: 1. Heparin
2. Low molecular weight heparins; Dalteparin, Enoxaprin
3. Warfarin

Action: They prevent clot formation and extension, do not dissolve clots.

Uses: Prevention and treatment of thromboembolic disorders; deep vein thrombosis, pulmonary embolism, atrial fibrillation with embolism, myocardial infarction.

Side Effects: Common side effects are: diarrhea, rash, fever, anemia, hepatitis. Serious side effects being: bleeding, thrombocytopenia, leukopenia.

General Nursing Considerations

- **Assess:** BP, Hb, Platelet, BT, PT, APTT, bleeding gums, petechia, ecchymosis, black tarry stools, hematuria, nose bleed, skin rash. Any unexplained fall in BP or hematocrit should lead to a search for a bleeding site
- **Administration:** Use infusion pump to deliver accurate dosage. For subcutaneous use, preferred site is abdominal wall above iliac crest, upper outer side of thigh, upper quadrant of buttock; rotate site; inject at an angle of 45° or 90°. It is given at same time each day to maintain steady blood levels. Apply pressure over injection and venipuncture sites to prevent bleeding or hematoma formation. Do not change brand. Do not rub site after injection. Keep vitamin K ready for emergency use. Avoid smoking, may increase dose requirements
- **Advise:** Avoid IM injections and hazardous activities. Use soft toothbrush and electric razor. Report bleeding and bruising
- **Desired Outcome:** Prevention of stroke, MI, deep vein thrombosis, pulmonary embolism.

1. Heparin

Dosage:

- Anticoagulation:
- Adults: IV: Intermittent: Initial 10,000 units, followed by 5000–10,000 units every 4–6 hours. Continuous: 5000 units initially, followed by 20,000–40,000 units over 24 hours. SC: 5000 units IV, followed by SC dose of 10,000–20,000 units, then 8000–10,000 units every 8 hours.

Children >1 year: Intermittent: 50–100 units/kg, then 50–100 units/kg every 4 hours.

Continuous: Initial 75 units/kg followed by 20 units/kg/hour.

- **Prevention of thromboembolism: Adults: SC: 5000 units every 8–12 hours**
- **Cardiovascular surgery: Adults: IV: 150 units/kg for procedure <60 minutes** and 400 units/kg if >60 minutes
- Line flushing: Adults and Children: Use 10–100 units/mL solution to fill heparin lock set upto needle hub.

Brands: 1000 and 5000 units/mL Inj; Beparin, Heparin.

Nursing Consideration: It can be given IV undiluted or diluted in 250–500 mL of normal saline or D_5W and given at the required rate.

2. Low Molecular Weight Heparins—Dalteparin, Enoxaparin

Dosage:

- Dalteparin: Adults: SC:

  Prevention of deep vein thrombosis following abdominal surgery: 2500 units 1–2 hours before surgery, then once daily for 5–10 days. Unstable angina: 120 units/kg every 12 hours for 5–8 days with aspirin
- Enoxaparin:

  Adults: SC: Treatment of deep vein thrombosis/pulmonary embolism: 1 mg/kg every 12 hours. Unstable angina: 1 mg/kg every 12 hours for 2–8 days. Prevention of deep vein thrombosis in abdominal surgery: 40 mg once daily for 7–10 days

  Children >2 months <18 years: SC: Prophylaxis 0.75 mg/kg every 12 hours and for treatment 1 mg/kg every 12 hours; subsequent doses are titrated as required.

Brands: Dalteparin: 2500 and 5000 units/0.2 Inj; Fragmin. Enoxaparin: 20 mg/0.2 ml Inj; Clexane, Lupenox.

3. Warfarin

Dosage:

- Adults: PO, IV: 2.5–10 mg/day for 2–4 days, later dosage are adjusted as per PT values
- Children >1 month: PO, IV: Initial dose of 0.2 mg/kg for 2–4 days, later dosage are adjusted as per PT values.

Brands: 1, 2, 5 mg Tabs; Uniwarfin, warf.

Nursing Consideration: For IV dilute 5 mg in 2.7 ml of sterile water and infuse over 2–3 minutes.

Chapter 10

Anticonvulsants

Includes: (A) Barbiturates (B) Benzodiazepines (C) Hydantoins (D) Valproates (E) Miscellaneous

These agents are used for seizures and epilepsy. Some agents are also used for other indications.

General Nursing Considerations

- **Assess:** BP, HR, LFT, RFT, CBC, PT, EEG, serum electrolytes periodically. Seizures duration, type, frequency, location. Respiratory status, level of sedation, mood, memory, pain; duration, site, frequency
- **Administration:** Give round the clock to maintain steady blood level and effect. Abrupt withdrawal may precipitate status epilepticus. Some drugs may lead to physical and psychological dependence on chronic use. During IV use monitor closely for respiratory depression and cardiovascular collapse. Supplement vitamin D to prevent hypocalcemia and folic acid to prevent megaloblastic anemia
- **Advise:** Avoid activities requiring alertness, smoking, alcohol and other CNS depressants. Avoid dangerous activities (driving, crossing road alone, standing at sea/river edge, bright light exposure, high levels, etc.). They should be advised to be taken at fixed time each day. Combine psychotherapy to decrease anxiety, exercise, relaxation techniques; along with drugs. Maintain good oral hygiene, use soft toothbrush, massage gums. Report rash, fever, severe headache, pain in mouth
- **Desired Outcome:** Decrease or cessation of seizures.

(A) ANTICONVULSANTS—BARBITURATES

Include: 1. Phenobarbital 2. Thiopental

Action: Decreases neuron excitability, raises seizure threshold.

Side Effects: Common side effects are; drowsiness, hangover, lethargy, respiratory depression. Serious effects include; serum sickness, angioedema, laryngospasm.

1. Phenobarbital

Uses: GTCS, PS, FS, neonatal seizures, sedation.

Dosage

- Anticonvulsant: IV: loading dose
  Neonates: 15–20 mg/kg in single or divided doses
  Adults and Children: 15–18 mg/kg in single or divided doses
- Anticonvulsant: IV, PO: Maintenance dose (start 12 hours after loading dose)
  Neonates: 3–4 mg/kg/day once daily
  Adults and Children: 5–6 mg/kg/day in 1–2 divided doses
- Sedation
  Adults: PO, IM: 30–100 mg/day in 2–3 divided doses
  Children: PO: 2 mg/kg, 3 times/day.

Brands: 30, 60 mg Tabs; 20 mg/5 ml Syp; Gardenal. 200 mg/mL Inj. Phenobarb.

Nursing Consideration: IV can be given at the rate of 1 mg/kg/min, with maximum of 30 mg/min for children and 60 mg/min for adults.

2. Thiopental

Uses: Convulsions, sedation, induction of anesthesia.

Dosage: IV

- Anesthesia induction: Adults and Children >12 years: 3–5 mg/kg. Children 1–12 years: 5–6 mg/kg
- Anesthesia maintenance: Adults: 12–100 mg as needed. Children: 1 mg/kg as needed
- Convulsions: Adults: 75–250 mg/dose, repeat as needed
  Children: 2–3 mg/kg/dose, repeat as needed.

Brands: 500, 1000 mg/mL Vial; Anesthal, Repantenal.

Nursing Consideration: IV can be given over 10–60 minutes at a maximum concentration of 50 mg/mL. Extravasation may cause tissue necrosis.

(B) ANTICONVULSANTS—BENZODIAZEPINES

Include:
1. Clobazam
2. Clonazepam
3. Diazepam
4. Lorazepam
5. Midazolam

Action: Depresses all levels of the CNS, presynaptic inhibition for anticonvulsant effects. Diazepam also causes skeletal muscle relaxation.

Side Effects: Drowsiness, lethargy, ataxia, behavioral changes, orthostatic hypotension, respiratory depression.

1. Clobazam

Uses: Anxiety, epilepsy.

Dosage: PO

- Adults: 20–30 mg/day single or in divided doses
- Children: 100–200 μg/kg twice daily.

Brands: 5, 10, 20 mg Tabs; Cloba, Frisium.

2. Clonazepam

Uses: Absence, akinetic, myoclonic seizures; infantile spasms, panic disorder.

Dosage: PO: Administer with food.

- Anticonvulsant: Adults and Children ≥10 years: 0.5 mg, 3 times/day
  Children <10 years: 0.01–0.03 mg/kg/day (Max: 0.05 mg/kg/day)
- Panic disorder: Adolescents and adults: 0.25 mg twice daily.

Brands: 0.5, 1, 2 mg Tabs; Lonazep, Melzep.

3. Diazepam

Uses: Anxiety, sedation, panic disorders, status epilepticus, as skeletal muscle relaxant.

Dosage:

- Anxiety: Adults: PO: 2–10 mg, 2–4 times/day. IM, IV: 2–10 mg, 3–4 times/day
  Children: PO: 0.04–0.3 mg/kg/dose, 3–4 times as needed
- Sedation: Adults: IM: 10 mg before surgery
  Children: PO: 0.2–0.3 mg/kg, 45–60 minutes before procedure
- Status epilepticus: Adults: IV: 5–10 mg every 10–15 minutes to a total dose of 30 mg
  Children: 1 month–5 years: 0.05–0.3 mg/kg/dose given over 3–5 minutes, every 15–30 minutes to max total dose of 5 mg
  Children ≥5 years: 0.05–0.3 mg/kg/dose (Max: 10 mg)
- Muscle relaxant: Adults: PO: 2–10 mg 2–4 times/day. IM, IV: 5–10 mg
  Children 1 month–5 years: IV, IM: 1–2 mg/dose every 3–4 hours as needed
  Children ≥5 years: IV, IM: 5–10 mg/dose every 3–4 hours as needed.

Brands: 2, 5 and 10 mg Tabs; 5 mg/mL Inj; Calmpose, Placidox.

Nursing Consideration: Rapid IV push may cause sudden respiratory depression, apnea or hypotension. IV should be given at the rate of 5 mg/min in adults and 1-2 mg/min in children.

4. Lorazepam

Uses: Anxiety, sedation, status epilepticus.

Dosage:

- Anxiety: Adults: PO: 1–3 mg, 2–3 times/day
  Children: PO, IV: 0.02–0.1 mg/kg/dose every 4–8 hours
- Status epilepticus: IV
  Adults: 4 mg/dose may be repeated in 10–15 minutes
  Children: 0.1 mg/kg slow IV over 2–5 minutes; may be repeated after 15 minutes in a dose of 0.05 mg/kg
  Neonates: 0.05 mg/kg over 2–5 minutes, may be repeated in 10–15 minutes

Brands: 1, 2 mg Tabs; 2 mg/mL Inj; Lopez, Loripam.

Nursing Consideration: IV can be given diluted in D_5W, Normal Saline (NS) in equal volume, at the maximum rate of 2 mg/min or 0.05 mg/kg over 2–5 minutes.

5. Midazolam

Uses: Anxiety, sedation, status epilepticus.

Dosage:

- Infants ≥2 months and children: Status epilepticus: IV: Loading dose of 0.15 mg/kg followed by continuous infusion of 1 μg/kg/minute (titrate dose)
- Infants >6 months and children: Sedation, anxiety: IM: 0.1–0.15 mg/kg 30–60 minutes before surgery or procedure. IV: 0.25–0.05 mg/kg (titrate dose)
- Adults: Sedation: IM: 0.07–0.08 mg/kg, 30–60 minutes before surgery. IV: 2.5–5 mg (titrate dose).

Brands: 1 and 5 mg/mL Inj; Mezolam, Midaz.

Nursing Consideration: Administer PO empty stomach. For IM maximum concentration is 1 mg/mL and for IV it is 5 mg/mL, and it should be given slowly over 2–5 minutes diluted in D5W or NS.

(C) ANTICONVULSANTS—HYDANTOINS

Include: 1. Fosphenytoin 2. Phenytoin

Action: Decreases seizure propagation by altering ion transport and stabilizes neuronal membranes. Phenytoin also have antiarrhythmic property by decreasing pacemaker automaticity and prolongs refractory period.

Side Effects: Common side effects being; ataxia, diplopia, nystagmus, dizziness, nausea, pruritus, gingival hyperplasia (phenytoin), hypotension. Serious side effects are; SJS, agranulocytosis, aplastic anemia.

1. Fosphenytoin

Uses: Status epilepticus, GTCS.

Dosage: Expressed as phenytoin equivalent (PE), 1.5 mg fosphenytoin = 1 mg phenytoin.

- Anticonvulsant: Adults: Loading dose: IV: 15–20 mg PE/kg. Maintenance dose: IV, IM: 4–6 mg PE/kg/day
  Children: Loading dose: IV: 10–15 mg PE/kg. Maintenance dose: IV, IM: 4–8 mg PE/kg/day.

Brands: 75 mg/mL Inj; Fosolin, Fosphen.

Nursing Consideration: IV should be diluted in NS or D5W to 1.5 mg/mL and given at the rate of 3 mg PE/kg/min.

2. Phenytoin

Uses: GTCS, SPS, CPS, antiarrhythmic.

Dosage:

- Status epilepticus: IV
  Adults and Children: Loading dose: 15–18 mg/kg single or divided doses Maintenance dose (Started 12 hours after loading dose). Adults: 4–6 mg/kg/day in 2–3 divided doses. Children: 6–8 mg/kg/day in 2 divided doses

- Anticonvulsant: PO
  Adults and Children: Loading dose: 15–20 mg/kg in 3 divided doses
  Maintenance dose: Same as IV maintenance dose
- Antiarrhythmic:
  Adults and Children: Loading dose: IV: 1.25 mg/kg every 5 minutes, may be repeated to total dose of 15 mg/kg
  Adults: Maintenance dose: PO: 300–400 mg/day in divided doses
  Children: Maintenance dose: PO, IV: 5–10 mg/kg/day in 2 divided doses.

Brands: 50, 100 mg Tabs; 25 mg/mL Inj. Epsolin.

Nursing Consideration: For IV dilute in NS, it can be given at the rate of 50 mg/min in adults and 1 mg/kg/min in pediatric patients followed by NS flushes to avoid local irritation. Maintain good oral and dental hygiene. Diabetic patients should monitor blood sugar levels.

(D) ANTICONVULSANTS—VALPROATES

Action: Increases levels of inhibitory neurotransmitter GABA in the CNS which decreases seizure activity.

Uses: Partial seizures, absence, mixed seizures, manic episodes.

Dosage:

- Seizures: Adults and Children: PO: Initial dose of 10–15 mg/kg/day in 1–3 divided doses, may be increased slowly up to max of 30–60 mg/kg/day as required
- Mania: Adults: PO: 750 mg/day in divided doses.

Brands: Valproate: 200, 300 mg Tabs; 200 mg/5 mL Syp; Valparin.
Divalproex sodium: 250, 500, 750 mg Tabs; Torvate.

Side Effects: Common side effects being; abdominal pain, nausea, vomitting, diarrhea, dizziness, insomnia, headache, sedation, tremor. Serious side effects are; hepatotoxicity, pancreatitis, hyperammonemia.

Nursing Consideration: Administer PO with meals at bedtime.

(E) ANTICONVULSANTS—MISCELLANEOUS

Include:

1. Acetazolamide
2. Carbamazepine
3. Gabapentin
4. Lamotrigine
5. Levetiracetam
6. Oxcarbazepine
7. Pregabalin
8. Topiramate
9. Zonisamide

1. Acetazolamide

Action: Acts by inhibition of carbonic anhydrase at various sites.

Uses: Adjunct to seizures, diuretic, raised intra/occular pressure, to decrease CSF production in hydrocephalus.

Dosage: PO

- Adults: Epilepsy: 4–16 mg/kg/day in 1–4 divided doses
  Glaucoma: 250–1000 mg/day in divided dose
  Edema: 250–375 mg/day once daily
- Children: Epilepsy: 4–16 mg/kg/day in divided doses
  Glaucoma: 8–30 mg/kg/day in divided doses
  Edema: 5 mg/kg/day once daily

Brands: 250 mg Tabs; Diamox, Acetamide.

Side Effects: Common side effects are; anorexia, weight loss, metallic taste, depression. Serious side effects include; SJS, hemolytic anemia, leukopenia.

Nursing Consideration: Watch for eye discomfort, signs of hypokalemia (muscle weakness, ECG changes, vomiting). Daily weight, input and output. PO with food. Supplement potassium if required.

2. Carbamazepine

Action: Decreases sodium influx across membrane resulting in decreased synaptic transmission.

Uses: GTCS, partial seizures, trigeminal neuralgia.

Dosage: PO

- Adults: Seizures: 200 mg twice daily (Max: 1200 mg/day)
  Neuralgia: 100 mg twice daily
- Children: 6–12 years: 100 mg twice daily (Max: 800 mg/day)
  <6 years: 10–20 mg/kg/day in 2 divided doses.

Brands: 100, 200, 400 mg Tabs; Mazetol, Tegretol. 100 mg/5 ml Syp; Mazetol

Side Effects: Common side effects are; hepatitis, drowsiness, ataxia, diarrhea. Serious side effects are; aplastic anemia, thrombocytopenia, SJS, hypertension.

Nursing Consideration: High fat meal may increase rate of absorption. PO with food.

3. Gabapentin

Action: Stabilizes neuronal membrane.

Uses: Partial seizures, postherpetic neuralgia.

Dosage: PO

- Seizures: Adults and Children >12 years: 300 mg, 3 times/day
  Children ≥3–12 years: 10–15 mg/kg/day in 3 divided doses
- Neuralgia: Adults: day 1–300 mg once; day 2–300 mg twice; day 3–onwards 300 mg thrice.

Brands: 100, 300, 400 mg Cap; Gabantin, Gabatin.

Side Effects: Ataxia, drowsiness, confusion, leukopenia.

Nursing Consideration: PO ± food. Antacids decreases bioavailability by 20%.

4. Lamotrigine

Action: Stabilizes neuronal membrane by decreasing sodium transport.

Uses: GTCS, partial seizures.

Dosage: PO: It can be given with or without food.

- No valproic acid: Adults and Children >16 years: 1st and 2nd week, 50 mg/day. 3rd and 4th week, 100 mg/day in 2 divided doses. Maintenance after 4 weeks 500 mg/day in 2 divided doses
- With valproic acid: Adults and Children: 25 mg/day for 1–4 weeks then 150 mg/day in divided doses

Brands: 25, 50, 100 mg Tabs; Lamepil.

Side Effects: Nausea, vomiting, abdominal pain, ataxia, headache, dizziness.

5. Levetiracetam

Uses: GTCS, partial and myoclonic seizures in adults.

Dosage:

- Adults: IV, PO: Initial dose of 500 mg once or twice daily, may be increased after 2 weeks (Max: 3000 mg/day)
- Children: 6–16 years: PO: 10 mg twice daily may be increased after 2 weeks interval (Max: 60 mg/kg/day)

Brands: 250, 500, 750 mg Tabs; 100 mg/mL Inj; Levroxa.

Side Effects: Somnolence, vertigo, ataxia, tremors, headache, diarrhea.

Nursing Consideration: Use IV only if PO use is not possible. PO ± meals. IV should be given diluted in 100 mL of NS/D_5W/RL over 15 minutes.

6. Oxcarbazepine

Action: Decreases propagation of synaptic impulses, blocks sodium channels of neuronal membranes.

Uses: Partial seizures.

Dosage: PO ± food.

- Adjunct therapy: Adults: 300 mg twice daily
  Children: 4–5 mg/kg twice daily
- Convertion to monotherapy: Adults: 300 mg twice daily
  Children: 8–10 mg/kg/day twice daily.

Brands: 150, 300, 600 mg Tabs; Oxcarb, Oxep.

Side Effects: Nausea, vomiting, abdominal pain, drowsiness, headache, diplopia, ataxia, tremor.

7. Pregabalin

Action: Binds to CNS calcium channels.

Uses: Partial seizures, pain due to postherpetic neuralgia and diabetic neuropathy.

Dosage: Adults: PO±meals.

- Seizures: Initially 150 mg/day in 2-3 divided doses, may be increased to maximum of 600 mg/day gradually
- Pain: Initially 50-75 mg twice daily (Max: 300 mg/day).

Brands: 75,100,150 mg Cap; Gabafit.

Side Effects: Vomiting, dry mouth, drowsiness, edema.

8. Topiramate

Uses: GTCS, partial seizures.

Dosage: Anticonvulsant: PO±food.

- Adolescents and adults: Initially; 25-50 mg/kg/day (Max: 200 mg BD)
- Children: 2-16 years: Initially; 1-3 mg/kg/day is divided doses (Max: 9 mg/kg/day)

Brands: 25,50,100 mg Tabs; Topamate.

Side Effects: Nausea, vomiting, fatigue, speech problem, ataxia, weight loss, diplopia.

Nursing Consideration: Increase fluid intake to more than 3 L/day to prevent stone formation. Change position slowly to prevent orthostatic hypotension.

9. Zonisamide

Uses: Partial seizures.

Dosage: PO: Adults and Children >16 years: Initially 100 mg twice daily for 2 weeks then 200 mg twice daily.

Brands: 25, 50, 100 mg Cap; Zonit.

Side Effects: Nausea, vomiting, drowsiness, fatigue.

Chapter 11 Antidepressants

Include: (A) Selective serotonin reuptake inhibitors (SSRTs)
(B) Tetracyclic
(C) Tricyclic
(D) Miscellaneous

These agents are used for treatment of various forms of depression. Some agents are used for multiple indications.

General Nursing Considerations

- **Assess:** Mental status, mood, worsening depression or suicidal tendencies specially in young patients, urinary retention, sexual dysfunction. BP, PR, weight, LFT, CBC. When using tricyclic drugs assess for tachycardia and increase in anginal attacks; they may precipitate MI or stroke
- **Administration:** Give sedating drug at bedtime and those causing insomnia in the morning. Give irritating drug with food to avoid gastric irritation. In adolescents and adults use lower initial doses than in adults
- **Advise:** Inform that effect may take 2–3 weeks to appear and combine psychotherapy along with medicine. Avoid alcohol and other CNS depressant drugs, activities requiring alertness. Change position slowly to avoid orthostatic hypotension. Increase fluid and fiber intake and exercises to prevent constipation. Maintain good oral hygiene and frequent oral rinses to decrease dry mouth sensation. It may cause drowsiness and dizziness. Taper the drug gradually as abrupt withdrawal may lead to side effects. Report hallucinations, blurred vision or excessive stimulation
- **Desired Outcome:** Decrease in depression, anxiety, chronic pain, increased sense of well-being, bedwetting as applicable to particular drug.

(A) ANTIDEPRESSANTS—SELECTIVE SEROTONIN REUPTAKE INHIBITORS (SSRIs)

Include:
1. Citalopram
2. Duloxetine
3. Escitalopram
4. Fluoxetine
5. Fluvoxamine
6. Paroxetine
7. Sertraline

Action: Inhibits reuptake of serotonin in the CNS.

Side Effects: Abdominal pain, anorexia, dry mouth, diarrhea, increased salivation and sweating, drowsiness, insomnia, weakness, tremors, sexual disturbances.

Nursing Consideration: Refer main discussion, Page no. 76.

1. Citalopram

Uses: Depression.

Dosage: Adults: PO: 20–40 mg/day either in the morning or evening.

Brands: 10, 20, 40 mg Tab; C-Talo, Citara, Madam.

2. Duloxetine

Uses: Depression, anxiety, diabetic neuropathic pain.

Dosage: Adults: PO

Depression: 20–30 mg 2 times/day. Anxiety and neuropathic pain: 60 mg once a day.

Brands: 20, 30, 40 mg Cap; Dulane, Dulot, Duxet.

3. Escitalopram

Uses: Depression, anxiety.

Dosage: Adults: PO: 10–20 mg once a day, either in morning or evening.

Brands: 5, 10, 20 mg Tab; Cilentra, Citofast.

4. Fluoxetine

Uses: Depression, OCD, bulimia nervosa.

Dosage: Adults: PO: Depression, OCD: 20–40 mg/day. Bulimia: 40–60 mg/day.

Children (7–17 years): PO: 10–20 mg/day.

Brands: 10, 20, 60 mg Cap; Fludac, Flunil.

Nursing Consideration: Given in 2 divided doses, one in the morning and second at noon time, ±food.

5. Fluvoxamine

Uses: OCD, depression, anxiety.

Dosage: PO: Start at lower doses and gradually increase the dose weekly.

- Adults: 50–100 mg/day at bedtime
- Children (8–17 years): 25–50 mg/day at bedtime

Brands: 50, 100 mg Tab; Fluvoxin, Ocivox, Sorest.

6. Paroxetine

Uses: Depression, OCD, anxiety, panic disorder.

Dosage: Adults: PO: Start at lower doses and increase it gradually.

- Depression, anxiety: 20–50 mg/day
- OCD, panic disorder: 20–40 mg/day.

Brands: 10, 20, 30 mg Tab; Pari, Xet.

7. Sertraline

Uses: Depression, panic disorder, OCD, anxiety.

Dosage: PO: Given in the morning or evening.

- Adults: Depression, OCD: 50–100 mg once a day.
  Panic disorder, anxiety: 50–100 mg once a day.
- Children: 6–12 years: OCD, 25 mg once a day.
  13–17 years: OCD, 50 mg once a day.

Brands: 25, 50, 100 mg Tab; Lindep, Serlift.

(B) ANTIDEPRESSANTS—TETRACYCLIC

Include: 1. Mianserin 2. Mirtazapine

Action: Blocks the reuptake of serotonin and norepinephrine into nerve endings.

Uses: Depression.

Side Effects: Dry mouth, constipation, increased appetite, weight gain, drowsiness, hypertension, seizures.

Nursing Consideration: Refer main discussion, page no. 76

1. Mianserin

Dosage: Adults: PO: 30–60 mg once a day at bedtime.

Brands: 10, 30 mg Tab; Depnon, Tetradep.

2. Mirtazapine

Dosage: Adults: PO: 15–45 mg once a day at bedtime.

Brands: 7.5, 15, 30 mg Tab; Mirpine, Mirtaz.

(C) ANTIDEPRESSANTS—TRICYCLIC

Include:
1. Amitriptyline
2. Clomipramine
3. Desipramine
4. Doxepin
5. Imipramine
6. Nortriptyline

Action: Potentiates the action of serotonin and norepinephrine in the CNS and also has anticholinergic properties.

Uses: Depression. Imipramine is also used for nocturnal enuresis and clomipramine for OCD.

Side Effects: Arrhythmias, constipation, drowsiness, sedation, hypotension, blurred vision, tachycardia, urine may discolor to blue-green.

Nursing Consideration: Refer main discussion, page no. 76

1. Amitriptyline

Dosage: PO

- Adults: 75–150 mg once a day at bedtime
- Adolescents: 25–100 mg once a day at bedtime.

Brands: 10, 25,75 mg Tab; Amitone, Tryptomer.

2. Clomipramine

Dosage: PO

- Adults: Antidepressant: 25 mg, 3 times/day. OCD: 25–100 mg/day in divided doses
- Children: >10–17 years: 25 mg 3 times/day.

Brands: 25, 50, 75 mg Tab; Clomip, Clonil.

3. Desipramine

Dosage: PO

- Adults: 100–200 mg/day divided every 12 hours
- Children: 6–12 years: 25–50 mg/day divided every 12 hours
  >12 years: 10–30 mg/day divided every 12 hours.

Brands: 10, 25, 75 mg Tab; Norpramin.

4. Doxepin

Dosage: PO: Adults: 25 mg, 3 times/day.

Brands: 10, 25, 75 mg Tab; Doxetor, Spectra.

5. Imipramine

Dosage: PO

- Adults: 25–50 mg, 3 or 4 times/day
- Children: Antidepressant: 6–12 years; 10–30 mg/day divided every 12 hours.
  >12 years; 25–50 mg/day divided every 12 hours.
  Enuresis: 25–50 mg at bedtime.

Brands: 25, 75 mg Tab; Antidep, Antipres.

Nursing Consideration: For enuresis give 1 hour before bedtime.

6. Nortriptyline

Dosage: PO

- Adults: 25 mg TDS
- Adolescents: 30–50 mg/day in divided doses.

Brands: 25 mg Tab; Nordep, Sensewal.

(D) ANTIDEPRESSANTS—MISCELLANEOUS

Include: 1. Amoxapine 2. Bupropion 3. Trazodone

1. Amoxapine

Uses: Depression.

Dosage: Adults: PO: 50 mg 2 or 3 times/day at bedtime.

Brands: 50,100 mg Tab; Demolox, Oxamine.

Side Effects: Refer tricyclic antidepressants, page no. 78

2. Bupropion

Action: Refer tricyclic antidepressants, page no. 78

Uses: Depression.

Dosage: Adults: PO: 100–150 mg, 2 or 3 times/day.

Brands: 150 mg Tab; Zyban.

Nursing Consideration: Refer main discussion, page no 76

3. Trazodone

Action: Alters effect of serotonin in the CNS.

Uses: Depression, insomnia.

Dosage: Adults: PO

- Depression: 150 mg/day in divided doses
- Insomnia: 25–100 mg at bedtime.

Brands: 25, 50, 100 mg Tab; Depryl, Traze.

Side Effects: Dry mouth, hypotension, drowsiness.

Nursing Consideration: Refer to main discussion, page no. 76

Chapter

12 Antidiabetics

Include: (A) Alpha glycoside inhibitors (B) Biguanides
(C) Meglitinides (D) Sulfonylureas
(E) Thiazolidinediones

These agents are used to control elevated blood glucose levels. Insulin is used for type I and oral hypoglycemic agents are used for type II DM. During pregnancy insulin is a recommended drug for controlling glucose level. Drugs control but does not cure DM and therapy is usually lifelong. Stable patient on diabetic regimen during fever, stress, infection, trauma or surgery may require additional insulin. Observe for signs and symptoms of hypoglycemia (sweating, tremors, dizziness, weakness, anxiety, tachycardia) and hyperglycemia (dry mouth, dry skin, drowsiness, fruit like breath odor, increased urination, nausea, vomiting, unconsciousness, rapid deep breathing). In event of hypoglycemia patient should carry sugar, glucose, honey or orange juice. Patient should strictly follow prescribed medicine, diet and exercise to avoid hypoglycemia and hyperglycemia. Patient and family should learn how to test blood glucose and urine ketones specially during stress and illness.

(A) ANTIDIABETICS—ALPHA GLYCOSIDE INHIBITORS

Include: 1. Acarbose 2. Miglitol

Action: Inhibits the enzyme alpha-glycoside in the GI tract, resulting in delayed glucose absorption and decreased blood glucose level.

Uses: Treatment of type II DM.

Side Effects: Diarrhea, abdominal pain, flatulence.

General Nursing Considerations

- **Assess:** Blood glucose, glycosylated Hb, LFT; signs and symptoms of hypoglycemia and hyperglycemia
- **Administration:** Along with first bite of each meal. These agents usually does not cause hypoglycemia when taken during fasting but may increase hypoglycemic effect of other agents
- **Desired Outcome:** Control of blood glucose level to near normal levels.

1. Acarbose

Dosage: Adults (PO): 25 mg, 3 times/day may be increased every 4 weeks up to 50–100 mg 3 times/day.

Brands: 25, 50 mg Tab; Diabose, Asucrose, Rebose.

Nursing Consideration: In event of hypoglycemia use oral glucose as sugar is not effective.

2. Miglitol

Dosage: Adults (PO): 25 mg, 3 times/day can be increased gradually upto 100 mg, 3 times/day.

Brands: 25, 50 mg Tab; Diamig, Miglit, Mignar.

Nursing Consideration: May experience abdominal pain and diarrhea which should diminish with continued use.

(B) ANTIDIABETICS—BIGUANIDES

Metformin

Action: Decreases intestinal glucose absorption, decreases hepatic glucose production, increases insulin sensitivity.

Uses: Treatment of type II DM.

Dosage: PO+meals.

- Adults: Initially 500 mg twice daily may be increased weekly (Max: 2000 mg/day)
- Children >10–17 years: 500 mg twice daily.

Brands: 250, 500, 750 mg Tab; Bigomet, Glyciphage, Glycomet.

Side Effects: Nausea, vomiting, abdominal bloating, hypoglycemia, signs of lactic acidosis.

Nursing Consideration:

- **Assess:** Blood glucose, glycosylated Hb, serum electrolytes, ketones, lactate, RFT; signs and symptoms of hypoglycemia
- **Administration:** Supplement vitamin B_{12} in patients on long-term therapy. Small dose with insulin therapy may enhance glucose control
- **Advise:** May cause lactic acidosis so watch for signs and symptoms of it (diarrhea, dyspnea, chills, BP, HR, dizziness). May cause metallic taste which resolves itself. Avoid alcohol, consume plenty of fluids
- **Desired Outcome:** Control of blood glucose level.

(C) ANTIDIABETICS—MEGLITINIDES

Include: 1. Nateglinide 2. Repaglinide

Action: Stimulates pancreatic insulin release.

Uses: Treatment of type II DM.

Side Effects: Diarrhea, dizziness, chest pain, symptoms of hypoglycemia.

Nursing Consideration: Assess blood glucose and glucosylated Hb, signs and symptoms of hypoglycemia. Take exactly as directed.

1. Nateglinide

Dosage: Adults: PO, 1/2–1 hour before meal. 120 mg, 3 times/day.

Brands: 60, 120 mg Tab; Glinate, Natelide, Notiz.

2. Repaglinide

Dosage: Adults: PO, 30 minutes before meal. 0.5–4 mg/day (Max: 16 mg/day).

Brands: 0.5, 1,2 mg Tab; Eurepa, Regon, Repide.

(D) ANTIDIABETICS—SULFONYLUREAS

Include: 1. Chlorpropamide 2. Glibenclamide 3. Gliclazide 4. Glimepiride 5. Glipizide 6. Tolbutamide

Action: Stimulates release of insulin from pancreas and increases receptor sensitivity to insulin.

Uses: Treatment of type II DM.

Side Effects: Diarrhea, hepatitis, dizziness, headache, hypoglycemia, photosensitivity, signs of aplastic anemia.

General Nursing Considerations

- **Assess:** Blood glucose, glycosylated Hb, CBC, LFT, RFT, signs and symptoms of hypoglycemia, allergy to sulfonamides
- **Administration:** Once daily in the morning with breakfast or divided daily in two doses
- **Advise:** Use sunscreen and protective clothing. Concurrent use of alcohol may cause disulfiram like reaction (abdominal pain, flushing, nausea, headache, hypoglycemia)
- **Desired Outcome:** Decrease in blood glucose level.

1. Chlorpropamide

Dosage: Adults (PO): 100–500 mg/day.

Brands: Chlorpropamide + Phenformin: 50 + 25 mg Tab; Chlorformin.

2. Glibenclamide

Dosage: Adults (PO): Initially 2.5–5 mg daily (Max: 15 mg/day in divided doses).

Brands: 2.5, 5 mg Tab; Aviglen, Daonil, Glycosafe.

3. Gliclazide

Dosage: Adults (PO): Initially 40–80 mg/day (Max: 320 mg/day).

Brands: 30, 40, 60, 80 mg Tab; Glizid, Nuzid, Reclide.

4. Glimepiride

Dosage: Adults (PO): Initially 1–4 mg once daily (Max: 8 mg/day).

Brands: 1, 2, 3, 4 mg Tab; Betaglim, Dibiglim, Novaride.

5. Glipizide

Dosage: Adults (PO): Initially 5 mg/day (Max: 40 mg/day).

Brands: 5, 10 mg Tab; Dibizide, Glynase.

6. Tolbutamide

Dosage: Adults (PO): 500–1000 mg, twice daily.

Brands: 500 mg Tab; Rastinone.

(E) ANTIDIABETICS—THIAZOLIDINEDIONES

Include: 1. Pioglitazone 2. Rosiglitazone

Action: Increases pancreatic insulin secretion and increases insulin sensitivity.

Uses: Treatment of type II DM.

Side Effects: Hepatitis, raised liver enzymes, edema, anemia, fractures in female. Rosiglitazone also causes CHF, lactic acidosis.

Nursing Consideration: Assess blood glucose, glycosylated Hb, CBC, LFT, RFT, signs and symptoms of hypoglycemia. Can be given per orally with or without food. Do not use in presence of hepatic dysfunction and CHF.

1. Pioglitazone

Dosage: Adults (PO): 15–30 mg once daily (Max: 45 mg/day).

Brands: 15, 30 mg Tab; Diavista, Pioglit, Piozed.

2. Rosiglitazone

Dosage: Adults (PO): 2 mg twice daily (Max: 4 mg twice daily).

Brands: 2, 4, 8 mg Tab; Enselin, Reglit, Rosicon.

Nursing Consideration: Assess for signs and symptoms of CHF (dyspnea, edema, crepitations, raised JVP, weight gain), signs of lactic acidosis (respiratory distress, malaise, muscle pain, abdominal discomfort, hypothermia, hypotension, bradyarrhythmias).

Chapter

13 Antidiarrheals

Include: 1. Diphenoxylate/Atropine
2. Loperamide
3. Racecadotril

Action: Diphenoxylate and loperamide act by slowing intestinal mobility and propulsion. Racecadotril only decreases hypersecretion.

Uses: Adjunctive therapy for acute and chronic nonspecific secretory diarrhea.

Side Effects: Common side effects are; constipation, nausea, dry mouth, abdominal pain, drowsiness. Serious side effects include; paralytic ileus and toxic megacolon.

General Nursing Consideration

- **Assess:** Fluid, electrolyte, dehydration status; frequency and consistency of stools; bowel sounds
- **Administration:** It should not be used as sole drug if there is associated fever or abdominal pain. In cases of acute diarrhea it should be used for only <48 hours, if no response seen then discontinue. In chronic cases if no improvement within 10 days then these drugs are unlikely to be effective
- **Advise:** Drink plenty of fluids to prevent dehydration, they may cause drowsiness so avoid activities requiring alertness. To reduce dry mouth sensations maintain good oral hygeine, use chewing gum
- **Desired Outcome:** Decrease in diarrhea.

1. Diphenoxylate + Atropine

Dosage: PO

- Adults: 5 mg 3–4 times/day initially, then 5 mg once daily as needed
- Children >2 years: 0.3–0.4 mg/kg/day divided every 6 hours

Brands: Diphenoxylate 2.5 mg+Atropine 0.025 mg tabs; Lomotil.

2. Loperamide

Dosage: PO

- Adults and Children ≥12 years: 4 mg initially, then 2 mg after each loose stool up to 8 mg/day

- Children: Initial dose: 2–5 years: 1 mg 3 times/day;
  6–8 years: 2 mg 2 times/day;
  8–12 years: 2 mg 3 times/day;

followed by 0.1 mg/kg doses after each loose stool but not to exceed initial dose.

Brands: 2 mg Tabs; 1 mg/5 ml liquid; Andial.

3. Racecadotril

Dosage: PO

Adults: 100–200 mg upto 3 times/day.

Children: 1.5 mg/kg 3 times/day.

Brands: 10, 30 mg Tabs; Zedott. 100 mg cap; 10, 30 mg sachet; Redotril, AD, Enuff.

Chapter

14 Antidotes/Poisoning

1. Acetylcysteine

Action: Mucolytic property, restores glutathione levels.

Uses: Antidote for acute acetaminophen toxicity.

Dosage:

- IV: Initially 150 mg/kg given over 15 minutes, followed by 50 mg/kg for over 4 hours, then 100 mg/kg over 16 hours
- PO: Initially 140 mg/kg, followed by 17 doses of 70 mg/kg every 4 hours.

Brands: 600 mg Tab; Mucomix. 200 mg/mL 20% solution; Mucare, Mucolyte, Mucomix.

Side Effects: Nausea, hemoptysis, drowsiness, bronchospasm, hypotension, tachycardia.

Nursing Consideration: For IV use dilute first dose in 200 mL of D_5W, second in 500 and third in 1000 mL of D_5W. Acute flushing and erythema may occur within 1/2–1 hour after IV infusion.

2. Bupropion

Action: Decreases neuronal uptake of dopamine, serotonin and norepinephrine.

Uses: Smoking cessation.

Dosage: PO ± food. 150 mg once daily for 3 days, then 150 mg twice daily for 7–12 weeks.

Brands: 150 mg Tab; Zyban.

Side Effects: Common side effects are; dry mouth, change in appetite, agitation, headache, tremor. Serious ones include; seizures.

3. Charcoal

Action: Adsorbent detoxicant.

Uses: Acute management of many oral poisoning and overdoses of certain drugs to enhance their excretion.

Dosage: PO

- Adults: 25–100 g (may be given every 6 hours)
- Children: 1–12 years: 25–50 g (may be given every 6 hours).
  <1 year: 1 g/kg (may be given every 6 hours).

Brands: 400 mg activated charcoal+80 mg simethicon Tab; Distenil.

Side Effects: Black stools, constipation, diarrhea, vomiting.

Nursing Consideration: It should only be given if patient is conscious. Most effective if given within 30 minutes of acute poisoning. If given along with milk or icecream it may reduce its effectiveness. Advise to drink slowly as rapid administration may increase vomiting.

4. Desferrioxamine

Action: Chelating agent.

Uses: Acute and chronic iron intoxication.

Dosage: IM, IV

- Acute iron ingestion: Adults and children ≥3 years: Initially 1 g, then 500 mg every 4 hours for 2 doses
- Chronic iron overload: Adults and children ≥3 years: 500 mg–1 g daily. Give additional 2 g for every unit of blood transfused.

Brands: 500 mg/Vial; Desferal.

Side Effects: Abdominal pain, red urine, blurred vision, hypotension, tachycardia, leg cramps.

Nursing Consideration: IM route is preferred over IV. Reconstitute 500 mg in 2 mL of SWI. This can be used for IM, for IV dilute it further and infuse at the rate of 15 mg/kg/hr. Rapid IV push may cause urticaria, hypotension and shock.

5. Dimercaprol

Action: Chelating agent.

Uses: Antidote to gold, arsenic, mercury poisoning.

Dosage: Adults and children (IM).

- Gold and arsenic poisoning: 2.5–3 mg/kg/dose every 4–6 hours for 2 days, then every 6–12 hours for 10 days
- Mercury poisoning: 5 mg/kg initially, followed by 2.5 mg/kg/dose 1–2 times/day for 10 days.

Brands: 100 mg/Vial; BAL.

Side Effects: Nausea, vomiting, tachycardia, fever, seizures, paresthesias.

Nursing Consideration: Administer IM undiluted.

6. Disulfiram

Uses: Management of chronic alcoholism.

Dosage: Adults (PO): 500 mg/day for 1–2 weeks, then 250 mg/day.

Brands: 500 mg Tab; Chronol. 250 mg Tab; Disulfiram.

Side Effects: Common side effects being; metallic taste, headache, drowsiness, optic neuritis, peripheral neuropathy. Serious one includes; hepatic toxicity.

7. Mesna

Action: Acts by binding to toxic metabolites of drugs.

Uses: Protection against hemorrhagic cystitis induced by ifosfamide and cyclophosphamide.

Dosage: Depends upon dose of antineoplastic agent used.

- Ifosfamide: Give mesna IV equal to 20% of dose of ifosfamide concurrently then 40% at 2 and 6 hours after ifosfamide
- Cyclophosphamide: Mesna dose is 20% of cyclophosphamide dose 15 minutes before and then every 3 hours for 3–4 doses.

Brands: 100 mg/mL Inj; Mesna, Uromes.

Side Effects: Unpleasant taste, vomiting, headache, flushing, flu-like symptoms, hypotension.

Nursing Consideration: Ensure adequate hydration before therapy. First dose is given as bolus, for subsequent doses dilute in D_5W/RL/NS to achieve a concentration of 20 mg/mL and infuse over 15–30 minutes.

8. Naloxone

Action: Competes and displaces narcotics at narcotic receptor sites.

Uses: Reversal of CNS and respiratory depression in suspected narcotic overdose.

Dosage: Postoperative opioid induced respiratory depression.

- Adults (IV): 0.02–0.2 mg every 2–3 minutes until response seen
- Children (IV): 0.01 mg/kg every 2–3 minutes until response seen
- Neonates (IM, IV, SC): 0.01 mg/kg every 2–3 minutes until response seen.

Brands: 200 and 400 µg/mL Inj; Narcoten. 400 µg/mL Inj; Nex.

Side Effects: Nausea, vomiting, hypertension, arrhythmias.

Nursing Consideration: Monitor RR, pulse, ECG, BP; level of consciousness; signs and symptoms of opioid withdrawal. For <40 kg dilute 0.1 mg in 10 mL of SWI/NS and infuse over 30 seconds.

9. Penicillamine

Action: Chelating agent, depresses circulating IgM rheumatoid factor level.

Uses: Heavy metal poisoning, Wilson's disease, rheumatoid arthritis.

Dosage: PO

- Wilson's disease: Adults: 250 mg 6 hourly. Children >6 months: 20 mg/kg/day in divided doses
- Antirheumatic: Adults: 125–250 mg/day as single dose. Children: 3 mg/kg/day for 3 months, then 6 mg/kg/day in 2 divided doses for 3 months.

Brands: 150, 250 mg Cap; Artamin.

Side Effects: Common side effects are; anorexia, altered taste, cholestatic jaundice, drug induced hepatitis. Serious side effects are; aplastic anemia, glomerulonephritis.

Nursing Consideration: Administer on empty stomach 1 hour before or 2 hours after meals, milk. Monitor CBC, urine, LFT.

10. Physostigmine

Action: Inhibits destruction of acetylcholine by acetylcholinesterase.

Uses: Reverses toxic CNS and cardiac effects caused by anticholinergics and TCAD.

Dosage:

Reversal of toxic anticholinergic effects

- Adults (IM, IV, SC): Initially 0.5-2 mg, repeat every 20 minutes until response or adverse effects seen
- Children (IV): Reserve for life-threatening situations only. 0.01–0.03 mg/kg/dose may repeat after 15–20 minutes to a maximum total dose of 2 mg.

Side Effects: Sweating, salivation, lacrimation. Rapid IV push may cause seizures, asystole.

Nursing Consideration: It can be given undiluted at a maximum rate of 0.5 mg/min in children or 1 mg/min in adults. Monitor HR and RR.

Brand: 1 mg/ml Inj. Eserine.

11. Pralidoxime

Action: Reactivates cholinesterase that had been inactivated.

Uses: Organophosphate poisoning; control of overdose of neostigmine, pyridostigmine.

Dosage:

- Organophosphate poisoning (IV, IM): Use in conjunction with atropine.
  Adults: 1-2 g, repeat in 1-2 hours if muscle weakness persist, then at 10–12 hours intervals if recurs.
  Children: 20–50 mg/kg/dose, repeat in 1-2 hours if muscle weakness persist, then at 10–12 hours intervals if recurs.
- Neostigmine and pyridostigmine overdoses: Adults (IV): 1-2 g followed by increment of 250 mg every 5 minutes.

Brands: 500 mg and 1 gm Vial; Clopam.

Side Effects: Nausea, headache, tachycardia, hypertension, rash, muscle rigidity, blurred vision.

Nursing Consideration: Reconstitute with 20 mL of SWI first then dilute in normal saline (NS) to achieve a concentration of 20 mg/mL and infuse over 15–20 minutes.

12. Succimer

Action: Chelating agent.

Uses: Treatment of lead poisoning (level >45 μg/dL).

Dosage: Adults and children (PO): 10 mg/kg every 8 hours for 5 days then reduce to 10 mg/kg every 12 hours for 2 weeks. Repeat the course after 2 weeks intervals.

Brands: 100mg Cap; Chemet

Side Effects: Nausea, vomiting, headache, cough, rash, thrombocytopenia.

Nursing Consideration: Ensure adequate patient hydration before therapy. Monitor CBC, LFT, lead levels.

Chapter 15

Antiemetics

Include: (A) 5-HT_3 Antagonists
(B) Phenothiazines
(C) Miscellaneous

(A) ANTIEMETICS—5-HT_3 ANTAGONISTS

Include: 1. Dolasetron 2. Granisetron
3. Ondansetron 4. Palonosetron

Action: These agents act by blocking the effects of serotonin at 5 HT_3 receptor sites centrally as well as peripherally on vagal nerve terminals.

Uses: Nausea and vomiting of various etiology including surgery, anesthesia, antineoplastic and radiation therapy. Palonosetron is specifically used for chemotherapy induced vomiting.

Side Effects: Common side effects are; headache, dizziness, hypotension, diarrhea, hypertension, extrapyramidal reactions, QTc interval prolongation, sedation, sleep disorders.

General Nursing Considerations

- **Assess:** Nausea, vomiting, bowel sounds, abdominal pain before and after therapy, input and output, hydration status. Patients with severe nausea and vomiting may require additional IV fluid therapy. Generally, if centrally mediated through CTZ, and there is nausea without vomiting, whereas if the vomiting center were triggered directly, then may see retching with vomiting. Ensure no obstruction of intestine and any drug overdose
- **Advise:** General measures to decrease nausea—small frequent sips of liquids, light diet, remove noxious stimuli from the immediate surroundings. Change position slowly to prevent orthostatic hypotension
- Ondansetron and Palonosetron may cause dry mouth.

1. Dolasetron

Dosage:

- Prevention or treatment of postoperative nausea and vomiting:
Administer PO 2 hours before and IV 15 minutes prior to surgery.
Adults (PO): 100 mg as a single dose. (IV): 12.5 mg as a single dose.

Children >2–16 years (PO): 1.2 mg/kg as a single dose (Max: 100 mg)
(IV): 0.35 mg/kg as a single dose (Max: 12.5 mg).

- Prevention of chemotherapy induced nausea and vomiting: Administer PO 1 hour before and IV 30 minutes prior to chemotherapy.
  Adults (PO): 100 mg as a single dose.
  (IV): 1.8 mg/kg as a single dose.
  Children >2–16 years (PO, IV): 1.8 mg/kg or alternatively 100 mg as a single dose.

Brands: 50, 100 mg Tabs; 10 mg/mL Susp; 20 mg/ml Inj; Anzemet.

Nursing Consideration

- **Monitor:** Vitals after IV use, as it may cause hypotension, bradycardia, syncope
- **Administration:** IV can be given undiluted in a concentration of 20 mg/mL over 1 minute. Compatible with NS/DNS/RL.

2. Granisetron

Dosage:

- Prevention and treatment of postoperative nausea and vomiting: Given prior to induction of anesthesia or just prior to reversal of anesthesia.
  Adults (IV): 1–2 mg as a single dose
  Children >4 years (IV): 20–40 μg/kg as a single dose (Max: 1 mg)
- Prevention and treatment of chemotherapy induced nausea and vomiting: First dose 1 hour before and second dose 12 hours later only on days when chemotherapy is given, for PO; and 30 minutes prior for IV use.
  Adults (PO): 2 mg once daily
  Adults and Children 2–16 years (IV): 10 μg/kg or 9 mg/day.

Brands: 1 mg Tabs; 1 mg/5 mL Syp; 1 μg/mL Inj; Grandem, Graset.

Nursing Considerations:

- **Assess:** Extrapyramidal symptoms (facial grimacing, rigidity, involuntary movements, trembling hands, shuffling walk)
- **Administration:** Infuse IV undiluted over 30 seconds or dilute in small volume of NS/D_5W and infuse for over 5 minutes.

3. Ondansetron

Dosage:

- Prevention of postoperative nausea and vomiting: IV, IM: Give immediately before induction of anesthesia or postoperatively.
  Adults and Children >40 kg: 4 mg as a single dose
  Children ≥2 years <40 kg: 0.1 mg/kg as a single dose
- Prevention of chemotherapy induced or radiotherapy induced nausea and vomiting: PO, IV:
  Adults and Children >12 years: 8 mg 3 times/day
  Children 4–11 years: 4 mg 3 times/day
  Children <4 years: 1–3 mg 3 times/day.

Brands: 4, 8 mg Tabs; 2 mg/5 mL Syp; 2 mg/mL Inj; Emeset, Periset, Ondem.

Nursing Consideration: Administer undiluted IV over 2–5 minutes or dilute in 50 mL of NS/DNS and infuse for over 15 minutes. Administer IM undiluted.

4. Palonosetron

Dosage: Adults: IV

Prevention of acute and delayed chemotherapy induced nausea and vomiting: 0.25 mg as a single dose (given 30 minutes prior and repeat dose within 7 days is not recommended).

Brands: 0.25 mg/5 mL Inj; Aloxi, Palzen.

Nursing Consideration: Administer undiluted over 30 seconds.

(B) ANTIEMETICS—PHENOTHIAZINES

Include: 1. Chlorpromazine
2. Prochlorperazine
3. Promethazine

Action: Acts on CTZ area to inhibit nausea and vomiting, alters effects of dopamine in the CNS, anticholinergic blocking activity.

Uses: Nausea and vomiting caused by surgery, anesthesia, antineoplastic and radiation therapy.

Side Effects: Common side effects are; constipation, dry mouth, blurred vision, dry eyes, photosensitivity, sedation, extrapyramidal reactions. Serious side effect is neuroleptic malignant syndrome.

General Nursing Consideration

For details also refer to 5-HT_3 antagonists (page no. 91). These drugs should be discontinued 48 hours before and should not be resumed for 24 hours following myelography, as these are known to lower seizure threshold. Use with caution in children with viral illness. Increase bulk food and fluids to minimize constipation. Don't stop abruptly. Extremes of temperature should be avoided, as these drugs are known to impair body thermostasis. Extrapyramidal reactions are more common in pediatric patient with acute illness and dehydration, so there is need to be careful in such cases. Urine may turn pink to reddish brown in color.

1. Chlorpromazine

Uses: Nausea and vomiting, hiccups, schizophrenia/psychoses.

Dosage:

- Psychoses/Schizophrenia:
  Adults: (PO): 30–200 mg/day divided every 6–12 hours
  (IM, IV): 25–50 mg initially and then increase gradually
  Children: (PO): 0.5–1 mg/kg dose every 4–6 hours
  (IM, IV): 0.5–1 mg/kg/dose every 6–8 hours

- Nausea and vomiting:
  Adults: (PO): 10–25 mg every 4–6 hours
  (IM, IV): 25–50 mg every 4–6 hours
  Children: (PO): 0.5–1 mg/kg/dose every 4–6 hours
  (IM, IV): 0.5–1 mg/kg dose every 6–8 hours.

Brands: 25, 50,100 mg Tabs; Clozine, Megatil. 25 mg/mL Inj; Cain, Megatil.

Nursing Consideration: Monitor extrapyramidal reactions and neuroleptic malignant syndrome. Give IV diluted to 1 mg/mL in normal saline (NS) at a rate of 1 mg/min.

2. Prochlorperazine

Uses: Nausea, vomiting, psychoses.

Dosage:

- Antiemetic:
  Adults: (PO): 5–10 mg 3–4 times/day
  (IM, IV): 2.5–10 mg as needed 4–6 hours
  Children: (PO): 0.4 mg/kg/day divided every 6–8 hours
  (IM, IV): 0.1–0.15 mg/kg/dose every 8–12 hours
- Antipsychotic:
  Adults: (PO): 5–10 mg 3–4 times/day
  (IM): 10–20 mg every 4 hours as needed
  Children 2–12 years: (PO): 2.5 mg 2–3 times/day
  (IM): 0.13 mg/kg/dose.

Brands: 5, 25 mg Tabs; Protil, Stemetil. 12.5 mg/mL Inj; Stemetil, Steminol.

Nursing Consideration: For IV dilute 1 mg/mL in RL, NS or Dextrose and infuse at a rate of 1–5 mg/min.

3. Promethazine

Uses: Nausea, vomiting, allergic conditions, motion sickness, sedative.

Dosage:

- Antiemetic: Adults (PO, IM, IV): 12.5–25 mg every 4–6 hours as needed. Children (PO, IM, IV): 0.25–1 mg/kg every 4–6 hours
- Antiallergic: Adults (PO): 6.25–12.5 mg, 3 times/day. (IM, IV): 25 mg as needed
- Motion sickness: Adults (PO): First dose of 25 mg 30 minutes–1 hour before departure, then every 8–12 hours as needed. Children (PO): 0.5 mg/kg 30 minutes before departure, then every 12 hours as needed.

Brands: 10,25 mg Tabs; Phenergan, Prometh. 5 mg/5 mL Syp; Phenergan, Phena kid. 25 mg/mL Inj; Phenergan.

(C) ANTIEMETICS—MISCELLANEOUS

Include: 1. Dimenhydrinate 2. Domperidone
3. Meclizine 4. Metoclopramide

1. Dimenhydrinate

Action: Competes with histamine for H_1-receptor sites and decreases vestibular stimulation.

Uses: Nausea, vomiting, motion sickness.

Dosage: PO

- Adults and Children >12 years: 50–100 mg every 4–6 hours
- Children: 2–5 years: 12.5–25 mg every 6–8 hours
  6–12 years: 25–50 mg every 6–8 hours

Brands: 50 mg Tabs; 15.6 mg/5 mL Syp; 50 mg/mL Inj; Draminate.

Side Effects: Common side effects are; dry mouth, drowsiness, constipation. Serious one is seizures.

Nursing Consideration: Also refer to 5-HT_3 antagonists (Page no 91). Administer 1–2 hours before conditions precipitating motion sickness. IV can be give undiluted over 2–5 minutes.

2. Domperidone

Action: Dopamine antagonist; prokinetic.

Uses: Nausea, vomiting and symtomatic treatment of non-ucler dyspepsia.

Dosage:

- Nausea and vomiting: Adults: 10–20 mg every 4–8 hours (Max: 80 mg/day)
- Children: 0.3 mg/kg/dose every 4-8 hours.
- Non-ulcer dyspepsia: Adults: 10–20 mg thrice daily.

Brands: 5–10 mg Tab; 1 mg/mL Susp; 10 mg/mL Drops; Domped, Domperon, Motinorm. 30 mg Tab; Domestal, Vomistop.

3. Meclizine

Action: Has antiemetic, antihistamine, anticholinergic action.

Uses: Motion sickness, vertigo.

Dosage: Adults and Children >12 years: PO.

- Motion sickness: 25–50 mg 1 hour before travel, may repeat in 24 hours
- Vertigo: 25–100 mg/day in divided dose.

Brands: Meclizine 25 mg+Vitamin B_6 50 mg Tabs; PNV.

Side Effects: Drowsiness, dry mouth, blurred vision.

4. Metoclopramide

Action: Blocks dopamine receptors at CTZ of CNS, stimulates motility of upper GI tract and accelerates gastric emptying.

Uses: Nausea, vomiting, GERD, postsurgical and diabetic gastric stasis.

Dosage:

- Antiemetic: Adults and Children (PO, IV): 1–2 mg/kg/dose every 2–4 hours
- GERD: Adults (PO, IM, IV): 10–15 mg 30 minutes before meals and at bedtime
  Infants and children (PO, IM, IV): 0.4–0.8 mg/kg/day divided every 6 hours

- Gastroparesis (PO, IV): 10 mg before each meal and at bedtime for 2–8 weeks.

Brands: 10 mg Tab; 5 mg/5 mL syp; 5mg/mL Inj; Maxeron, Perinorm. Reglan.

Side Effects: Sedation, headache. (Also refer Phenothiazines, Page no. 93).

Nursing Consideration: IV can be given diluted in NS, RL, D_5W in a concentration of 0.2 mg/mL and should be given over 15–30 minutes. For details also refer to phenothiazines, page no. 93.

Chapter

16 Antifungals

Include:
1. Amphotericin-B
2. Fluconazole
3. Griseofulvin
4. Itraconazole
5. Ketoconazole
6. Terbinafine
7. Voriconazole

Action: They inhibit cell wall synthesis and also increases cell membrane permeability.

Side Effects: Common side effects are: nausea, vomiting, diarrhea, rash. Serious side effects are; hepatotoxicity, SJS, anaphylaxis, toxic epidermal necrosis.

General Nursing Considerations

- **Assess:** BP, pulse, respiration, CBC, LFT, serum electrolyte, culture and sensitivity, CSF culture, input and output, weight, signs and symptoms of infection (vitals, sputum, lung sounds, assess oral mucosa, nail-beds, pharyngeal mucosa, scalp and skin)
- **Administration:** Do not give along with antacids or H_2 blockers
- **Advise:** Long-term therapy is required for full cure. Take exactly as directed even if signs and symptoms subsides. Report any signs and symptoms of hepatic dysfunction (nausea, vomiting, anorexia, pale stool, dark urine, jaundice). Notify unusual bleeding or bruising. They may cause dizziness and drowsiness, so avoid activities requiring mental alertness
- **Desired Outcome:** Resolution of signs and symptoms of infection (decrease fever, rash, malaise; negative culture and sensitivity; decrease in skin irritation and vaginal discomfort).

1. Amphotericin-B

Uses: Severe systemic infection and meningitis caused by candida, aspergillus and mucor species; visceral leishmaniasis. Liposomal amphotericin-B is useful in cases refractory to or intolerant to conventional therapy.

Dosage: Conventional Amphotericin-B is started in a test dose of 0.1 mg/kg/dose, to a maximum of 1 mg and given over 1 hour. If test dose is tolerated then therapeutic dose of 0.4 mg/kg can be given on the same day. The daily dose then can be increased in 0.25 mg/kg increaments to a dose of 1.5 mg/kg/day. Liposomal Amphotericin-B can be used in a higher doses upto 2.5–5 mg/kg/day.

Liposomal Amphotericin B: Emperic therapy in systemic infection—3 mg/kg/day as once daily infusion. Visceral leishmaniasis—Day 1 to 5, 3 mg/kg once and for day 14 and 21, 3 mg/kg once daily.

Brands: 50 mg/vial; Amfotex, Fungizone.

Nursing Consideration: Monitor vitals and for hypersensitivity reactions during test dose and during the first few hours of therapy.

2. Fluconazole

Uses: Oropharyngeal, esophageal and vaginal candidiasis; systemic candidiasis.

Dosage:

- Oropharyngeal and esophageal candidiasis (PO, IV): Given for 14 days in oropharyngeal and for 21 days in esophageal candidiasis.
  Adults: 200 mg on day 1, then 100 mg/day
  Children > 14 days: 6 mg/kg on day1, then 3 mg/kg/day
- Vaginal candidiasis (PO):
  Adults: 150 mg as single dose
- Systemic candidiasis: Given for 28 days (PO, IV):
  Adults: 400 mg/day for 1 day, then 200–800 mg/day
  Children > 14 days: 6–12 mg/kg/day.

Brands: 50 and 150 mg Tab; Flucos, Zocon. 2 mg/mL Inf; Syscan, Zocon.

Nursing Consideration: IV doses are given in a concentration of 2 mg/mL over 1–2 hours at the rate of 200 mg/hr.

3. Griseofulvin

Uses: Tinea infection of skin, hair, nails; caused by Microsporum, Epidermophyton or Trichophyton.

Dosage: PO + food or fatty meal.

- Adults: Microsize: 500–1000 mg/day in divided doses
  Ultramicrosize: 350–750 mg/day in divided doses
- Children: Microsize: 10–20 mg/kg/day in divided doses
  Ultramicrosize: 5–10 mg/kg/day in divided doses
- Duration of therapy: *T. corporis*: 2–4 weeks. *T. pedis*: 4–8 weeks
  T. capitis: 4–6 weeks. *T. unguium*: 3–6 months

Brands: 250 and 500 mg Tab; Dermonorm, Fluvin.

4. Itraconazole

Uses: Oropharyngeal and esophageal candidiasis; Aspergillosis, Blastomycosis, Onchomycosis.

Dosage: PO + meal.

- Oropharyngeal candidiasis: 200 mg/day once daily for 2 weeks
- Esophageal candidiasis: 100 mg/day once daily for 3 weeks
- Aspergillosis, Blastomycosis, Histoplasmosis: 200 mg/day twice daily for 2 days, then 200 mg once daily
- Children: General doses: 3–5 mg/kg/day once daily.

Brands: 100 mg Cap; Canditral, Itospar.

5. Ketoconazole

Uses: Candidiasis, oral thrush, blastomycosis, histoplasmosis. Topically for *T. corporis, T. cruris, T. versicolor*; Shampoo is used for dandruff.

Dosage:
- Adults: 200–400 mg/day once daily
- Children and infants: 3.3–6.6 mg/kg/day once daily
- Shampoo: Apply twice weekly for 4 weeks
- Topical: Apply once or twice daily.

Brands: 200 mg Tab; Fungizole, ketozole. 2% solution; Dandoff.

Nursing Consideration: PO+meal to decrease nausea and vomiting. Concurrent use of alcohol may cause a disulfiram like reaction (rash, nausea, headache, flushing, edema) and increase the risk of hepatotoxicity.

6. Terbinafine

Uses: Onchomycosis and T. capitis.

Dosage: PO±food.
- Adults: 250 mg/dose once daily (6 weeks for fingernail and 12 weeks for toenail infection)
- Children: 125–250 mg once daily for 6 weeks.

Brands: 250 mg Tab; Daskil, Fungotek.

7. Voriconazole

Uses: Systemic fungal infection, esophageal candidiasis, deep seated SSTI; abdominal and kidney infection; aspergillosis.

Dosage:
- Adults and children (IV): Initially 6 mg/kg/dose every 12 hours for 2 doses, then 4 mg/kg/dose every 12 hours.
- Adults and children (PO):
  Patients < 40 kg: Initially 200 mg every 12 hours for 2 doses, then 100 mg every 12 hours.
  Patients ≥ 40 kg: Initially 400 mg every 12 hours for 2 doses, then 200 mg every 12 hours.

Brands: 200 mg Tab; 200 mg/Vial; Voraze.

Nursing Consideration: PO given 1 hour before or 1 hour after meal. Monitor complete visual function in patients on chronic therapy and allergic reactions during parenteral use. For IV dilute in SWI in a concentration of 10 mg/mL, it is further diluted in NS/RL/D_5W to a concentration of 0.5–5 mg/mL and given at the rate of 3 mg/kg/hour.

Chapter

17 Antihistamines

Include:

1. Astemizole
2. Azatadine
3. Cetirizine
4. Chlorpheniramine
5. Clemastine
6. Cyproheptadine
7. Desloratidine
8. Dimenhydrinate
9. Diphenhydramine
10. Fexofenadine
11. Hydroxyzine
12. Levocetirizine
13. Loratidine
14. Meclizine
15. Promethazine

Action: These agents compete with histamines for H_1 receptor sites. Most agents also have anticholinergic properties. Cyproheptadine also blocks the serotonin effects which leads to increased appetite.

Uses: Treatment of seasonal and perennial allergic rhinitis; chronic urticaria. Cyproheptadine as appetite stimulant. Dimenhydrinate and meclizine in addition also used as antiemetic and diphenhydramine as antitussives.

Side Effects: Drowsiness, headache, thickening of respiratory secretions, urinary retention, GI discomfort, dry mouth, blurred vision.

General Nursing Considerations

- **Assess:** Input and output; CBC on long-term use; BP, pulse; allergic symptoms (rhinitis, conjunctivitis, hives), lung sounds, type of respiratory secretions
- **Administration:** Inject IM preparations irritating to tissues deep into the muscle. Stop 2–4 days prior to skin testing to avoid false-negative results. For motion sickness, take 30–60 minutes before travel time
- **Advise:** Maintain fluid intake of 1500–2000 mL/day to decrease viscosity of respiratory secretions. Avoid activities requiring mental alertness. Avoid concurrent use of alcohol and other CNS depressants. Maintain good oral hygiene, frequent oral rinses to decrease dry mouth sensation
- **Desired Outcome:** Decrease in allergic symptoms, pruritus, anxiety; prevention or decrease in nausea, vomiting, motion sickness, vertigo as applicable to particular drug.

1. Astemizole

Dosage: PO, 1 hour before or 2 hours after meals.
- Adults and children >12 years: 10 mg OD
- Children 6–12 years: 5 mg OD.

Brands: 10 mg Tab; 5 mg/5 mL Syp; Astelong, Stemiz.

2. Azatadine

Dosage: PO
- Adults: 1–2 mg BD
- Children: 6–12 years; 0.5–1 mg 2 times/day. 1–6 years; 0.25 mg 2 times/day.

Brands: 10 mg Tab; 5 mg/5 mL Syp; Zadine.

3. Cetirizine

Dosage: PO ± food.
- Adults and Children >6 years: 5–10 mg/day
- Children: 1–5 years: 2.5–5 mg/day
- Children 6–12 months: 2.5 mg/day.

Brands: 5 and 10 mg Tab; Allercet. 5 mg/5 mL Syp; Alerid, Zyncet.

4. Chlorpheniramine

Dosage: PO+food.
- Adults: 4 mg 6 hourly
- Children: 6–12 years: 2 mg 6 hourly.

Brands: 4 mg Tab; Cadistin. 0.5 mg/5 mL Syp; Polaramine.

Nursing Consideration: Use with caution in patients with asthma. Young patients may be more susceptible to side effects and CNS stimulation.

5. Clemastine

Dosage: PO+food.
- Adults and children ≥12 years: 1–2 mg base 2 or 3 times/day
- Children 6–12 years: 0.5–1 mg base 2 times/day
- Infants and children <6 years: 0.25–0.5 mg base/day in divided doses.

Brands: 1 mg Tab; 0.1 mg/mL Syp; Tavegyl.

6. Cyproheptadine

Dosage: PO+food.
- Adults: 4 mg every 8 hourly.
- Children >2 years: 2–4 mg every 8–12 hourly.

Brands: 2 and 4 mg Tab; 2 mg/5 mL Syp; Ciplactin.

Nursing Consideration: Monitor food intake and weight routinely.

7. Desloratidine

Dosage: PO±food.

- Adults and children ≥12 years: 5 mg once a day
- Children: 6–11 years: 2.5 mg once a day
- Children: 2–5 years: 1.25 mg once a day.

Brands: 5 mg Tab; 2.5 mg/5 mL Syp; Rodera.

8. Dimenhydrinate

For details refer—antiemetics—miscellaneous (Chapter 15, page no. 94).

9. Diphenhydramine

For details refer—antitussives (Chapter 27, page no. 134).

10. Fexofenadine

Dosage: PO+food.

- Adults and children ≥12 years: 60 mg 2 times/day or 180 mg once a day
- Children: 2–11 years: 30 mg BD
- Children 6 months–2 years: 15 mg BD.

Brands: 30, 120 and 180 mg Tab; 60 mg/5 mL Syp; Allegra.

11. Hydroxyzine

For details refer—Antianxiety—miscellaneous (Chapter 4, page no. 20).

12. Levocetirizine

Dosage: PO

- Adults and children ≥12 years: 2.5–5 mg/day
- Children: 6–11 years: 2.5 mg once a day

Brands: 5 mg Tab; 2.5 mg/5 mL Syp; 1-AL, Airitis.

13. Loratidine

Dosage: PO±food.

- Adults and children ≥6 years: 10 mg once a day
- Children 2–5 years: 5 mg once a day.

Brands: 10 mg Tab; 5 mg/5 mL Syp; Alaspan, Loridin.

14. Meclizine

For details refer—antiemetics—miscellaneous (Chapter 15, page no. 94)

15. Promethazine

For details refer—antiemetics—phenothiazines (Chapter 15, page no. 93).

Chapter

18 Antihypertensives

Include:

(A) ACE inhibitors (B) Adrenergics
(C) Centrally acting antiadrenergics (D) Peripherally acting antriadrenergics
(E) Angiotensin receptor antagonists (F) Beta blockers
(G) Calcium channel blockers (H) Diuretics
(I) Vasodilators

These agents are used to treat hypertension of various etiology. Oral treatment is used for long-term control and parenteral therapy for hypertensive emergencies. Goal of therapy is to decrease BP to near normal levels and prevent end organ damage. These medicines can control but cannot cure hypertension. Encourage them to use additional methods of lowering BP (weight reduction, regular exercise, stopping smoking and alcohol, low sodium diet, stress control therapy). Teach patient and family how to check BP and pulse.

(A) ANTIHYPERTENSIVES—ACE INHIBITORS

Include: 1. Captopril 2. Enalapril 3. Lisinopril
4. Perindopril 5. Ramipril

Action: They act by blocking the convertion of angiotensin I to angiotensin II which is a vasoconstrictor.

Side Effects: Common side effects are; nausea, vomiting, taste disturbances, abdominal pain, drowsiness, headache, hypotension, cough, erectile dysfunction, proteinuria, hyperkalemia, flushing. Serious side effects include; angioedema, agranulocytosis.

General Nursing Considerations

- **Assess:** CBC, LFT, RFT, serum electrolytes, urine protein, BP, pulse, daily weight, signs and symptoms of CHF (dyspnea, JVP, peripheral edema, crepitations), signs of angioedema (dyspnea, facial puffiness)
- **Administration:** First dose may cause rapid fall in BP during initial few hours and this can be corrected by volume expansion. Correct hypovolemia before starting therapy. Withdraw diuretics 2–3 days prior to starting ACE inhibitors. It is contraindicated in bilateral renal artery stenosis. Do not give drug and diet containing potassium.

- **Advise:** Take exactly as directed even if feeling well. They may cause drowsiness, avoid activities requiring mental alertness. Change position slowly to avoid orthostatic hypotension. May cause persistent dry cough which will last till therapy and taste impairment which will gradually resolves over 8–10 weeks. Avoid excessive perspiration, vomiting, diarrhea, dehydration; may cause low BP.
- **Desired Outcome:** Decrease in BP and signs and symptoms of CHF and hypertension.

1. Captopril

Uses: Treatment of HT, CHF; improves survival in post MI patients.

Dosage: PO on empty stomach 1 hour before or 2 hours after meal.

- Adults: 12.5–25 mg 2–3 times/day
- Older children: 6.25–12.5 mg/dose every 12–24 hours
- Children: 0.3–0.5 mg/kg/dose in 2–4 divided dose
- Infants: 0.15–0.3 mg/kg/dose divided every 6 hours.

Brands: 12.5 and 25 mg Tab; Aceten, Capotril.

Nursing Consideration: Use lowest effective dose in patient with sodium and water depletion, on diuretic therapy and CHF. Long-term therapy may cause zinc deficiency, supplement it. Avoid potassium-rich diet.

2. Enalapril

Uses: Treatment of HT, CHF.

Dosage: PO±food.

- Adults: Initially 2.5–5 mg/day, increase as required
  Usual dose for HT: 10–40 mg/day divided every 12 hours
  Usual dose for CHF: 5–20 mg/day divided every 12 hours
- Infants and children: Initially 0.1 mg/kg/day divided every 12 hours, can be titrated upto maximum of 0.5 mg/kg/day.

Brands: 2.5, 5, 10 mg Tab; Dilvas, Envas, Minipril.

Nursing Consideration: It may take weeks for full hypotensive effect.

3. Lisinopril

Uses: Treatment of HT, CHF; improves survival in post MI patients.

Dosage: PO±food.

- Adults: HT: 10 mg once daily, can be increased gradually to maximum of 20–40 mg/day. CHF: 5 mg/day once daily (along with diuretics and digitalis)
- Children ≥ 6 years: Initially 0.07 mg/kg once daily (Max: 5 mg/day)

Brands: 2.5, 5, 10 mg Tab; Acinopril, Linvas, Liscard.

4. Perindopril

Uses: Treatment of HT, CHF.

Dosage: Adults (PO): 4 mg once daily may be increased slowly upto 16 mg/day in divided doses.

Brands: 2, 4 mg Tab; Covergyl, Perigard.

5. Ramipril

Uses: Treatment of HT, CHF.

Dosage: Adults (PO): 1.25 mg initially. Maintenance dose in 2.5-5 mg/day.

Brands: 1.25, 2.5, 5, 10 mg Tab; Hopace, Cardace, Ramicard.

(B) ANTIHYPERTENSIVES—ADRENERGICS

Clonidine

Action: Stimulates α_2 adrenergic receptors in the CNS causing decrease in vasomotor tone and heart rate.

Uses: Management of mild to moderate hypertension.

Dosage: PO±food. More effective if combined with diuretics.

- Adults: Initial 0.1 mg twice daily. Maintenance dose: 0.2-1.2 mg/day in 2-3 divided doses
- Children: 5-10 μg/kg/day divided every 8-12 hourly

Brands: 100 μg Tab; Arkamin. 150 μg Tab; Catapres.

Side Effects: Constipation, dry mouth, drowsiness, insomnia, palpitation, withdrawal phenomenon, respiratory depression.

Nursing Consideration:

- **Assess:** BP, pulse, ECG, blood sugar, input and output; daily weight, edema
- **Administration:** Give last dose of the day at bedtime to ensure overnight control of BP. Tolerance may develop on long-term use; an increased dose or addition of diuretics may improve response
- **Advise:** Take same time each day. Do not stop abruptly, taper gradually over 1 week. It may cause drowsiness. Change position slowly.

(C) ANTIHYPERTENSIVES—CENTRALLY ACTING ANTIADRENERGICS

Methyldopa

Action: Stimulates CNS alpha-adrenergic receptors resulting in decrease in BP and peripheral resistance.

Uses: Management of moderate to severe hypertension.

Dosage:

- Adults (PO): 250-500 mg 2-3 times/day. (IV): 250-500 mg every 6 hours
- Children (PO): 10 mg/kg/day divided every 8 hours. (IV): 5-10 mg/kg every 6 hours.

Brands: 250 mg Tab; Aldopam, Alphadopa, Sembrina.

Side Effects: Dry mouth, diarrhea, sedation, edema, urine discoloration, drug induced hepatitis.

Nursing Consideration:

- **Assess:** BP, pulse, input and output, daily weight, edema, LFT, RFT, CBC, serum sodium and potassium, PT
- **Administration:** PO±food, give doses increase in the evening to minimize sedation. For IV dilute in 100 mL of D_5W/NS/RL to achieve a concentration of ≤10 mg/mL and infuse over 30-60 minutes
- **Advise:** Take exactly as directed. May cause drowsiness. Drug tolerance may develops after 1-2 months of therapy.

(D) ANTIHYPERTENSIVES—PERIPHERALLY ACTING ANTIADRENERGICS

Include: 1. Doxazosin 2. Prazosin 3. Terazosin

Action: Inhibits postsynaptic alpha-adrenergic receptors causing venous and arteriolar dilatation. Also decreases smooth muscle contraction in prostatic capsule.

Uses: Treatment of mild to moderate hypertension, symptomatic treatment of Benign Prostatic Hypertrophy (BPH).

Side Effects: Constipation, dry mouth, dizziness, headache, blurred vision, flushing, first dose orthostatic hypotension, palpitation, sexual dysfunction, arthralgia.

General Nursing Considerations

- **Assess:** BP, pulse every 2-4 hours during first dose, syncope, input and output, daily weight, edema, symptoms of prostatic hyperplasia (urinary hesitancy, frequency, dysuria, urgency, dribbling)
- **Administration:** First dose may cause orthostatic hypotension (manifested by syncope, weakness, dizziness). So first dose may be given at bedtime to minimize this. Do not stop abruptly
- **Advise:** Take exactly as directed. May cause drowsiness. Change position slowly to avoid orthostatic hypotension. For BPH control; no fluid intake 4 hours before bedtime; empty bladder before going to bed; avoid alcohol and caffeine
- **Desired Outcome:** Decrease in BP and urinary symptoms.

1. Doxazosin

Dosage: PO ± food.

Adults: 1 mg once daily.

Brands: 1, 2, 4 mg Tab; Doxacard, Duracard.

2. Prazosin

Dosage: PO ± food.

- Hypertension: Adults: 1 mg 2-3 times/day.
  Children: 0.05-0.4 mg/kg/day divided every 8 hours
- Benign Prostatic Hypertrophy: Adults: 1-5 mg twice daily.

Brands: 2.5 and 5 mg Tab; Minipress XL gits. 1 and 2 mg Tab; Prazopress.

3. Terazosin

Dosage: Adults: PO ± food.

- Hypertension: 1 mg initially can be increased gradually upto 5 mg/day
- Benign Prostatic Hypertrophy: 1 mg at bedtime.

Brands: 1, 2, 5 mg Tab; Hytrin, Teralfa, Terapress.

(E) ANTIHYPERTENSIVES—ANGIOTENSIN RECEPTOR ANTAGONISTS

Include: 1. Candesartan 2. Irbesartan 3. Losartan 4. Telmisartan 5. Valsartan

Action: Blocks effect of angiotensin II at receptor sites.

Uses: Treatment of HT, CHF, diabetic nephropathy.

Side Effects: Abdominal pain, diarrhea, drug induced hepatitis, dizziness, headache, hypotension, edema, hyperkalemia, angioedema.

General Nursing Considerations

- **Assess:** BP, pulse, LFT, RFT, serum electrolytes, CBC, daily weight, signs and symptoms of CHF (edema, dyspnea, JVP, crepitations), signs of angioedema (facial puffiness, dyspnea)
- **Administration:** PO ± food
- **Advise:** Take exactly as directed. It may cause drowsiness. Change position slowly to avoid orthostatic hypotension. Avoid foods containing high levels of sodium and potassium. Avoid activities that may lead to reduction in fluid volume, i.e. excessive perspiration, vomiting, diarrhea, dehydration, it may cause low BP.
- **Desireed Outcome:** Decrease in BP and decreased progression of diabetic nephropathy.

1. Candesartan

Dosage: Adults (PO): Initially 4–16 mg once daily (Max: 32 mg/day).

Brands: 4, 8, 16 mg Tab; Candelona, Ipsita.

2. Irbesartan

Dosage: Adults (PO): Initially 150 mg once daily (Max: 300 mg/day).

Brands: 150, 300 mg Tab; Irovel, Xarb.

3. Losartan

Dosage: Adults (PO): Initially 50 mg once daily (Max: 100 mg/day).

Brands: 25, 50 mg Tab; Alsartan, Losar, Nusar.

4. Telmisartan

Dosage: Adults (PO): Initially 40 mg once daily (Max: 80 mg/day).

Brands: 20, 40 mg Tab; Tazloc, Telma, Telpres.

5. Valsartan

Dosage: Adults (PO): Initially 80 mg daily (Max: 160 mg/day).

Brands: 40, 80, 160 mg Tab; Valent, Valzaar.

(F) ANTIHYPERTENSIVES—BETA-BLOCKERS

Include:	1. Atenolol	2. Bisoprolol	3. Carvedilol
	4. Labetolol	5. Metoprolol	6. Nebivolol
	7. Pindolol	8. Propranolol	9. Timolol

Action: Blocks stimulation of β_2 adrenergic receptors.

Side Effects: Common side effects are; Diarrhea, liver dysfunction, fatigue, weakness, insomnia, blurred vision, erectile dysfunction, muscle cramps, bronchospasm. Serious side effects include; CHF, bradycardia, pulmonary edema, arrhythmias.

General Nursing Considerations

- **Assess:** BP, pulse, ECG, RFT, serum electrolytes, blood glucose, input and output, daily weight, signs and symptoms of CHF (dyspnea, JVP, crepitations, edema)
- **Administration:** PO±food. Take pulse before giving drug, if HR < 50/min or if arrhythmia occurs withhold therapy. May mask signs and symptoms of hypoglycemia, so do regular blood sugar examination
- **Advise:** Take exactly as directed. Avoid abrupt withdrawal as it may precipitate, HT, MI, arrhythmias. May increase sensitivity to cold. Rise slowly from lying position, dress warmly during cold weather, avoid excess of alcohol, tea, coffee
- **Desired Outcome:** Decrease in BP.

1. Bisoprolol

Uses: Treatment of HT.

Dosage: Adults (PO): 5 mg once daily (Max: 20 mg/day).

Brands: 2.5, 5, 10 mg Tab; Bisbeta, Cadrol, Corbis.

2. Carvedilol

Uses: Treatment of HT, CHF.

Dosage: Adults (PO): HT: 6.25 mg twice daily. CHF: 3.125 mg twice daily.

Brands: 3.125, 6.25, 12.5 mg Tab; Cardivas, Carvedil, Cevas.

3. Nebivolol

Uses: Treatment of HT.

Dosage: Adults (PO): 5 mg once daily.

Brands: 2.5 and 5 mg Tab; Nebert, Nevol, Nubeta.

4. Pindolol

Uses: Treatment of HT.

Dosage: Adults (PO): 5 mg twice daily.

Brands: 10, 15 mg Tab; Visken.

5. Timolol

Uses: Treatment of HT, prevention of Myocardial Infarction (MI) and migraine headache.

Dosage: Adults (PO): 10 mg twice daily.

* For details of Atenolol, Labetalol, Metoprolol, Propranolol refer to antianginal drugs (Chapter 3).

(G) ANTIHYPERTENSIVES—CALCIUM CHANNEL BLOCKERS

Include: 1. Amlodipine 2. Diltiazem 3. Felodipine 4. Nifedipine 5. Verapamil

1. Amlodipine

Action: Inhibits transport of calcium into myocardial and vascular smooth muscle cells.

Uses: Treatment of hypertension, angina pectoris.

Dosage: Adults (PO): 5–10 mg once daily.

Brands: 2.5, 5, 10 mg Tab; Amcard, Amlogard, Amlovas.

Side Effects: Nausea, gingival hyperplasia, dizziness, headache, edema, bradycardia, hypotension, flushing.

Nursing Consideration:

- **Assess:** BP, pulse, ECG, signs of CHF
- **Administration:** PO ± food. Do not stop suddenly
- **Advise:** Take as directed. It may cause drowsiness. Maintain good oral hygiene to prevent gingival hyperplasia. Change position slowly. Avoid prolonged standing, excessive heat, alcohol
- **Desired Outcome:** Decrease is BP and angina.

* For details of Diltiazem, Felodipine, Nifedipine, Verapamil refer to antianginal drugs (Chapter 3).

(H) ANTIHYPERTENSIVES—DIURETICS

For details refer to diuretics (Chapter 32).

(I) ANTIHYPERTENSIVES—VASODILATORS

Include: 1. Hydralazine 2. Sodium nitroprusside

1. Hydralazine

Action: Causes peripheral arteriolar vasodilation.

Uses: Treatment of moderate to severe hypertension.

Dosage: PO, given with meal for better absorption.
- Adults: Initially 10 mg twice/day (Max: 200 mg/day)
- Children: Initially 0.75–1 mg/kg/day divided every 6 hours

Brands: 10 mg Tab; Nepresol.

Side Effects: Nausea, vomiting, headache, sodium retention, tachycardia, peripheral neuropathy, SLE like syndrome.

Nursing Consideration:
- **Assess:** BP, pulse, CBC, electrolytes, LE cell preparation, daily weight, edema
- **Advise:** Take exactly as advised. May cause drowsiness and orthostatic hypotension
- **Desired Outcome:** Decrease in BP.

2. Sodium Nitroprusside

Action: Cause peripheral venous and arteriolar vasodilation.

Uses: HT crises, controlled hypotension during anesthesia.

Dosage: Adults and children (IV): Initially 0.3 µg/kg/min (Max: 10 µg/kg/min).

Brands: 50 mg/mL Vial; Pruside, Niside.

Side Effects: Nausea, abdominal pain, dizziness, headache, blurred vision, phlebitis, dyspnea, cyanide toxicity.

Nursing Consideration:
- **Assess:** BP, pulse, ECG, bicarbonate, PCO_2, pH, serum methemoglobin level
- **Administration:** For IV use dilute 50 mg in 250–500 mL of D_5W to achieve a concentration of 50–200 µg/mL. Prepared solution should be used within 24 hours and bottle should be covered with aluminium foil
- **Desired Outcome:** Decrease in BP.

Chapter

19 Antimigraine Drugs

Include: (A) Alpha-adrenergic Blockers
(B) 5-HT_1 Agonists

These agents are used for acute treatment of migraine headaches. These should be given at the first sign of headache. These agents should only be used during a migraine attack and are meant for relief of attacks but cannot prevent or decrease the number of attacks. Lying in a quiet, darkened room along with medication further help relieve headache. Assess pain frequency, location, duration and characteristics (nausea, vomiting, visual disturbances, phonophobia). Avoid smoking and alcohol which may precipitate or aggravate migraine headache. These drugs may cause dizziness or drowsiness, so avoid activities requiring mental alertness.

(A) ANTIMIGRAINE DRUGS—ALPHA-ADRENERGIC BLOCKERS

Include: 1. Dihydroergotamine 2. Ergotamine

Action: Stimulates alpha-adrenergic and 5-HT receptors causing vasoconstriction of dilated blood vessels.

Uses: Treatment of acute attack of migraine headache with or without aura, cluster headaches.

Side Effects: Common side effects are; abdominal pain, altered taste, diarrhea, hypertension, dizziness, muscle pain, numbness or tingling of fingures or toes. Serious one is Myocardial Infarction (MI).

General Nursing Considerations

- **Assess:** Pain, BP, peripheral pulses, signs of ergotism (nausea, vomiting, cold, numbness of fingers and toes, muscle weakness)
- **Administration:** Administer at the first sign of prodromal symptoms
- **Advise:** Avoid cold and report immediately any tightness or chest discomfort, change in heart rate (HR)
- **Desired Outcome:** Relief of headaches.

1. Dihydroergotamine

Dosage: Adults (IM, SC): Initially 1 mg; repeat 1 mg in 1 hour if required (Max: 3 mg/day or 6 mg/week). IV: Initially 0.5 mg may be repeated in 1 hour (Max: 2 mg/day or 6 mg/week).

Brands: 1 mg/mL Inj; DHE, Migranil.

Nursing Consideration: IV given undiluted over 1–2 minutes.

2. Ergotamine

Dosage: Adults (PO): Initially 1–2 mg then 1–2 mg every 30 minutes until attack subsides or total dose of 6 mg is given.

Brands: Tab. Migril (Ergotamine 2 mg+Cyclizine 50 mg + Caffeine 100 mg per tablet). Tab. Vasograin (Ergotamine 1 mg + Caffeine 100 mg + Paracetamol 250 mg + Prochlorperazine 2.5 mg per tablet).

Nursing Consideration: It should not be used for more than twice a week and there should be a gap of 5 days.

(B) ANTIMIGRAINE DRUGS—5-HT$_1$ AGONISTS

Include: 1. Rizatriptan 2. Sumatriptan

Action: Acts as an agonist at selective 5-HT$_1$ receptors causing vasoconstriction in intracranial blood vessels.

Uses: Treatment of acute migraine headaches.

Side Effects: Common side effects are; dry mouth, dizziness, drowsiness, weakness, chest pain. Serious side effects include; MI, coronary artery vasospasm.

General Nursing Considerations

- **Assess:** BP, pulse, ECG
- **Administration:** Administer as soon as symptoms of migraine attack appear, but can be given at any time during an attack. If symptoms return then second dose can be given. Keep a gap of 1–2 hours between two doses
- **Advise:** Reduce dose if propranolol is prescribed concurrently. Do not take within 24 hours of any other medicines used to treat headache or depression. May experience rebound headache if taken more than 2–3 times/week.

1. Rizatriptan

Dosage: Adults: PO with water: Initially 5–10 mg may be repeated in 2 hours (Max: 3 doses/day).

Brands: 5, 10 mg Tab; Rizact, Rizatan.

Nursing Consideration: Do not take rizatriptan within 24 hours of taking other vascular headache suppressants.

2. Sumatriptan

Dosage: Adults (PO): Initially 25 mg, may be repeated in 24 hours if required (Max: 300 mg/day). SC: Initially 6 mg, may repeat after 1 hour (Max: 12 mg/day).

Brands: 25, 50, 100 mg Tab; 6 mg/0.5 mL Inj; Suminat, Sumitre.

Chapter

20 Antiobesity Drugs

Include: 1. Fenfluramine 2. Orlistat 3. Rimonabant 4. Sibutramine

Action:

- Fenfluramine and Sibutramine: It decreases appetite by enhancing seratonergic transmission in the hypothalamus
- Orlistat: It is a lipase inhibitor that decreases absorption of the dietary fat
- Rimonabant: Blocks cannabinoid receptors in the brain and peripheral tissue and decreases appetite

Uses: Obesity management along with dietary and exercise therapy. Specially useful in patients with Diabetes Mellitus (DM), Hypertension (HT) and hyperlipidemia.

General Nursing Considerations

- **Assess:** BP, HR, blood sugar, weight and dietary intake before and during therapy, history of cholestasis, eating disorders, thyroid dysfunction
- **Administration:** Supplement multivitamins which should be taken after meals
- **Advise:** Take medicines for HT, DM and hyperlipidemia if coexisting. Follow calorie restriction, exercise, maintain mobility as advised
- **Desired Outcome:** Gradual weight loss.

1. Fenfluramine

Dosage: Adults: PO: 40–60 mg once daily with meals.

Brands: 20 mg Tabs; 40 mg Cap; Flabolin.

Side Effects: Dry mouth, diarrhea, depression.

2. Orlistat

Dosage: Adults and Children ≥16 years: PO: 60–120 mg 3 times/day with each meal containing fat.

Brands: 120 mg Cap; Obelit, Zerofat.

Side Effects: Fecal incontinence, oily evacuation and spotting, increased defecation.

Nursing Consideration: Supplement vitamin D, E, K and beta carotene. Psyllium can be added to decrease GI side effects. If there is no fat in the meal, then omit dose.

3. Rimonabant

Dosage: Adults: PO: 20 mg once daily in the morning before breakfast.

Brands: 20 mg Tabs; Zerofat-R.

4. Sibutramine

Dosage: Adults: PO 10 mg once daily.

Brands: 5, 10 mg Cap; Obego, Sibutrim.

Side Effects: Insomnia, dry mouth, constipation, seizures, anorexia.

Chapter

21 Antiparkinson Agents

Include: (A) Anticholinergic (B) Antiviral
(C) Dopamine agonists (D) MAO inhibitors

These agents are used for Parkinson's disease. Same are used for multiple indications.

General Nursing Considerations

- **Assess:** BP, pulse, RR, CBC, LFT, input and output; mental status, akinesia, tremor, rigidity, muscle spasms, drooling, shuffling gait, before and during therapy.
- **Administration:** Avoid abrupt withdrawal to prevent withdrawal symptoms. Give with food to decrease GI discomfort. Advise patient to remain supine during and after first dose of bromocriptine to avoid sudden fall in BP.
- **Advise:** Take exactly as advised. Change position slowly to minimize orthostatic hypotension. Avoid activities requiring alertness. Maintain good oral hygiene, frequent rinses to decrease dry mouth sensation. Increase fluid, bulky food and do exercise to prevent constipation. Avoid concurrent CNS stimulants. It decreases perspiration, so patient should be advised to remain indoor in cool environment to prevent over heating. Patient on levodopa therapy should avoid multivitamins.
- **Desired Outcome:** Decrease in tremor, rigidity, twitching; improvement in balance and gait; increase in mood, decrease in galactorrhea and restless leg; improved sleep; as applicable to particular drug.

(A) ANTIPARKINSON AGENTS—ANTICHOLINERGIC

Trihexyphenidyl

Action: Acts by blocking or competing at central acetylcholine receptors.

Uses: Parkinsonism.

Dosage: Adults (PO): Initially 1–2 mg/day, increase gradually to maintenance dose of 6–10 mg/day in divided doses.

Brands: 2 mg Tab; Arkane, Pacitone, Triphen.

Side Effects: Common side effects are; nausea, dry mouth, constipation, blurred vision, mydriasis, nervousness, headache, hypotension.

Nursing Consideration: Refer main discussion (as above).

(B) ANTIPARKINSON AGENTS—ANTIVIRAL

Amantadine

Action: Potentiates dopamine action in the CNS, prevents release of viral nucleic acid into host cell.

Uses: Parkinsonism, prophylaxis and treatment of influenza A viral infection.

Dosage: PO

- Parkinsonism: Adults: 100 mg BD (Max: 400 mg/day)
- Influenza: Adults and children >12 years: 100–200 mg 2 times/day
  Children 10–12 years: 100 mg 2 times/day
  Children 1–9 years: 5 mg/kg/day divided every 12 hours (Max: 150 mg/day).

Brands: 100 mg Cap; Amentrel, Comantrel.

Side Effects: Common side effects are; hypotension, mottling, ataxia, insomnia, edema, nausea, vomiting, urinary retention.

Nursing Consideration: If causing insomnia it should be given 4 hours before sleep. Full benefit may take 2 weeks of therapy. For more details refer to main discussion.

(C) ANTIPARKINSON AGENTS—DOPAMINE AGONISTS

Include:
1. Bromocriptine
2. Cabergolin
3. Carbidopa/levodopa
4. Pramipexole
5. Ropinirole

Action: Decarboxylation to dopamine or by activation of dopamine receptors. Cabergolin and bromocriptine also inhibits prolactin secretion.

Nursing Consideration: Refer to main discussion.

1. Bromocriptine

Uses: Parkinsonism, hyperprolactinemia, acromegaly.

Dosage: Adults (PO) + food.

- Parkinsonism: Initially 1.25 mg BD, can be increased every 2–4 weeks (Max: 100 mg/day)
- Hyperprolactinemia: Initially 1.25–2.5 mg/day, increased every 3–7 days (Max: 7.5 mg/day)
- Acromegaly: 1.25–2.5 mg/day for 3 days, can be increased every 3–7 days (Max: 30 mg/day).

Brands: 1.25, 2.5 mg Tab; Criptal, Proctinal.

Side Effects: Common side effects are; nausea, hypotension, dizziness, rash. Serious side effects include; MI, shock, convulsions.

Nursing Consideration: Give at bedtime to prevent dizziness and orthostatic hypotension. Therapeutic effect may take 2 months. For more details refer to main discussion.

2. Cabergolin

Uses: Parkinsonism, hyperprolactinemia.

Dosage: Adults (PO) ± food. 0.25 mg twice weekly may be increased monthly to maximum of 1 mg twice weekly.

Brands: 0.5, 1 mg Tab; Comforte.

Side Effects: Common side effects are; constipation, dizziness, headache, anorexia.

Nursing Consideration: Once the normal prolactin level is maintained for 6 months, drug may be tapered off. Give at bedtime to prevent orthostatic hypotension. For more details refer to main discussion.

3. Carbidopa/levodopa

Uses: Parkinsonism.

Dosage: Adults (PO) + food. 10 mg Carbidopa + 100 mg levodopa 3–4 times/day or 25 mg Carbidopa + 100 levodopa 3 times/day may be increased every 2 days (Max: 100 Carbidopa + 1000 mg levodopa).

Brands: 10+100, 25+100, 25+250 mg, Carbidopa + levodopa; Tab. Duodopa, LCD, Pardopa.

Side Effects: Common side effects are; nausea, vomiting, involuntary movements, hypotension, cardiac arrhythmias.

Nursing Consideration: May darken urine and sweat. Eyelid and muscle twitching may suggest toxicity. Therapeutic effect may take 2–3 weeks to occur. Limit protein intake with drug. For more details refer main discussion.

4. Pramipexole

Uses: Parkinsonism, restless leg syndrome.

Dosage: Adults (PO) + food.

- Parkinsonism: Initially 0.125 mg 3 times/day then may be increased weekly (Max: 4.5 mg/day in divided doses)
- Restless leg syndrome: Initially 0.125 mg once a day, 3 hours before bedtime may be increased weekly (Max: 0.5 mg).

Brands: 0.125, 0.25, 1 mg Tab; Miraprex.

Side Effects: Common side effects are; constipation, dry mouth, dyspepsia, nausea, amnesia, hallucinations, EPS, hypotension. Serious side effects include; sleep attacks, leukopenia.

Nursing Consideration: Refer main discussion.

5. Ropinirole

Uses: Parkinsonism, restless leg syndrome.

Dosage: Adults (PO) + food.

- Parkinsonism: Week 1, 0.25 mg 3 times a day; week 2, 0.5 mg 3 times a day; week 3, 0.75 mg 3 times a day; week 4, 1 mg 3 times a day; then can be increased weekly upto maximum of 3 mg 3 times a day
- Restless leg syndrome: Initially 0.25 mg once a day, 2–3 hours before bedtime. May be increased after 2 days and then weekly (Max: 4 mg/day).

Brands: 0.5, 1, 2 mg Tabs; Parkirop, Ropitor.

Nursing Consideration: Refer main discussion.

(D) ANTIPARKINSON AGENTS—MAO INHIBITORS

Selegiline

Action: Increases dopamine activity by inhibiting MAO type B activity.

Use: Parkinsonism.

Dosage: Adults (PO): 5 mg 2 times/day with breakfast and lunch.

Brands: 5 mg Tab; Eldepryl, Selgin.

Side Effects: Common side effects are; nausea, hypotension, edema.

Chapter

22 Antiplatelet Agents

Include: 1. Eptifibatide 2. Clopidogrel 3. Dipyridamole 4. Ticlopidine 5. Tirofiban

Action:

- Eptifibatide and Tirofiban decreases platelet aggregation by inhibiting glycoprotein II b/III a
- Dipyridamole decreases platelet aggregation by inhibiting phosphodiesterase enzyme and inhibit adenosine uptake to cause coronary vasodilatation
- Clopidogrel and Ticlopidine decreases platelet aggregation by inhibiting binding of ATP to platelet.

General Nursing Considerations

- **Assess:** BP, HR, ECG, input and output, LFT, RFT, bleeding, BT, PT, symptoms of stroke, MI, peripheral vascular disease, chills, fever
- **Administration:** Use infusion pump for IV use. If platelet count <1 lakh inform doctor. Avoid NG tube, urinary catheters and nasotracheal intubation. Required to be discontinued before surgery
- **Advise:** Report for any bleeding. Change position slowly to minimize postural hypotension. Avoid alcohol and tabacco. Brush teeth with soft bristle toothbursh, use electric razor for shaving, wear shoes while ambulating. Family should learn CPR
- **Desired Outcome:** Prevention of stroke, MI, vascular morbidity and mortality.

1. Eptifibatide

Uses: Unstable angina.

Dosage: Adults: IV: 180 μg/kg as bolus, followed by 2 μg/kg/minute for up to 72 hours.

Brands: 2 mg and 0.75 mg/mL Inj; Antigrilin, Coromax.

Side Effects: Bleeding, hypotension, thrombocytopenia.

Nursing Consideration: It can be given undiluted at the rate of 0.5–1 mL/minute.

2. Clopidogrel

Uses: MI, stroke, peripheral arterial disease.

Dosage: Adults: PO: 75 mg once daily.

Brands: 75 mg Tabs; Clavix, Clopitab.

Side Effects: Bleeding, headache, cough, dyspnea.

3. Dipyridamole

Uses: Coronary insufficiency, prophylaxis of thrombosis in patient of prosthetic heart valve.

Dosage:
- Adults: PO: 200–400 mg/day in divided doses
- Children: PO: 3–6 mg/kg/day in divided doses.

Brands: 25, 75, 100 mg Tabs; Cardiwell.

4. Ticlopidine

Uses: Prevention of stroke, ischemic heart disease, intermittent claudication.

Dosage: Adults: PO: 250 mg twice daily with food.

Brands: 250 mg Tabs; Ticlantin, Ticlop.

5. Tirofiban

Uses: Unstable angina.

Dosage: Adults: IV: 0.4 μg/kg/minute for 30 minutes, then 0.1 μg/kg/min as required for 24–48 hours.

Brands: 5 mg/100 mL Inj; Aggritor, Tirofuse.

Side Effects: Bleeding, headache, sweating, nausea.

Chapter

23 Antipsychotics

Includes: (A) Phenothiazines (B) Miscellaneous

(A) ANTIPSYCHOTICS—PHENOTHIAZINES

Include:
1. Chlorpromazine
2. Fluphenazine
3. Prochlorperazine
4. Thioridazine
5. Trifluoperazine

Action: Alters release and turnover of dopamine, blocks dopamine receptors; also has anticholinergic/alpha-adrenergic blocking activity.

Side Effects: Common side effects are; sedation, dry mouth, constipation, hypotension, dry eyes, blurred vision, photosensitivity. Serious side effects includes; agranulocytosis, laryngospasm, NMS, seizures.

General Nursing Considerations

- **Assess:** BP, pulse, RR, input and output, CBC, LFT, mental status, monitor for EPS, muscle spasms, twitching, difficulty in speaking or swallowing, fever, respiratory distress, tachycardia, convulsions, uncontrolled rhythmic movements
- **Administration:** PO with food or liquid to decrease GI irritation. May raise seizure threshold so it should be discontinued 48 hours prior and avoid for 24 hours after myelography. Keep supine for 30 minutes after parenteral dosing to avoid hypotensive crisis. Avoid other CNS depressants concurrently. Do not use pink or discolored solution
- **Advise:** Take exactly as directed. Avoid abrupt withdrawal to minimize withdrawal symptoms. Avoid activities requiring mental alertness. Increase bulk, fluid and activity to decrease constipation; maintain good oral hygiene and frequent oral rinses to minimize dry mouth. Change position slowly to avoid postural hypotension. These drugs impair temperature regulation, so avoid hot weather and hot showers. Report if excessively active or depressed. May discolor urine pink or reddish brown
- **Desired Outcome:** Decrease in excitement, delusions, hallucinations, relief in intractable hiccups and nausea, vomiting as applicable to particular drug.

1. Chlorpromazine

For details refer to antiemetic—phenothiazines and main discussion.

2. Fluphenazine

Uses: Schizophrenia.

Dosage:
- As Decanoate, adults (IM): 12.5–100 mg/day in divided doses
- As Hydrochloride, adults (IM): 1.25–2.5 mg every 6–8 hours.

Brands: 25 mg/mL Inj.; Anatensol, Fludecan.

3. Prochlorperazine

For details refer to antiemetic—phenothiazines and main discussion.

4. Thioridazine

Use: Schizophrenia.

Dosage: PO
- Adults and children > 12 years: 50–100 mg 3 times/day
- Children 2 ≤ 12 years: 0.5 mg/kg/day in divided doses.

Brands: 10, 25, 50 mg Tab; Melozin, Ridazin, Thioral.

5. Trifluoperazine

Uses: Schizophrenia, anxiety.

Dosage:
- Adults (PO): Psychoses; 2–5 mg 2 times/day. Anxiety; 1–2 mg 2 times/day. (IM): 1–2 mg every 4–6 hours.
- Children 6–12 years (PO, IM): 1 mg once a day or 2 times/day.

Brands: 5, 10 mg Tab; Neocam, Trinicalm.

(B) ANTIPSYCHOTICS—MISCELLANEOUS

Include:
1. Aripirazole
2. Clozapine
3. Haloperidol
4. Lithium
5. Olanzapine
6. Paliperidone
7. Quetiapine
8. Risperidone
9. Ziprasidone

1. Aripirazole

Action: Dopamine and serotonin antagonist, also has alpha-adrenergic blocking activity.

Uses: Schizophrenia, mania.

Dosage:
- Schizophrenia: Adults (PO): 10–20 mg/day once a day. (IM): 5–10 mg/day once a day. Children 13–17 years (PO): 2–10 mg/day once a day.
- Mania: Adults (PO): 30 mg once a day. (IM): 5–10 mg/day.

Brands: 10, 15, 20, 30 mg Tab; Arena, Aria, Arzu.

* For side effects and nursing considerations refer to phenothiazines.

2. Clozapine

Uses: Schizophrenia.

Dosage: Adults (PO): 25–300 mg/day; increase weekly.

Brands: 25, 50, 100 mg Tab; Lozapin, Sizopin, Skizoril.

* For side effects, action and nursing considerations refer to phenothiazines.

3. Haloperidol

Uses: Schizophrenia, mania, Tourette's syndrome.

Dosage:

- Adults (PO): 0.5–5 mg 2 or 3 times/day. (IM): 2–5 mg 3 times/day. (IV): 0.5–5 mg, may be repeated every 30 minutes.
- Children 3–12 years (PO): 50–75 µg/kg/day in divided doses.

Brands: 0.25, 1.5, 5 mg Tab; 50 mg/mL Inj; Depidol, Serance, Senorm.

* For action, side effects and nursing consideration refer to phenothiazines.

4. Lithium

Action: Alters neuronal uptake of neurotransmitters and cation transport in nerve and muscles.

Uses: Manic episodes of manic depressive illness.

Dosage: (PO): Monitor serum lithium levels.

- Adults and children ≥12 years: 300–600 mg 3 times/day
- Children <12 years: 15–20 mg/kg/day divided every 8 hours.

Brands: 300, 400 mg Tab; Carbolith, Licab.

Side Effects: Common side effects are; abdominal pain, diarrhea, anorexia, polyurea, headache, fatigue, hypothyroidism, tremor, muscle weakness. Serious side effects are; arrhythmias, seizures.

* For NC refer phenothiazines.

5. Olanzapine

Uses: Schizophrenia, mania.

Dosage: Adults (PO)

- Schizophrenia: 5–10 mg/day. Mania: 10–15 mg/day.

Brands: 2.5, 5, 7.5, 10, 15 mg Tab; Meltolan, Olace, Oleanz.

* For action, side effects and nursing consideration refer phenothiazines.

6. Paliperidone

Use: Schizophrenia.

Dosage: Adults (PO): 6 mg/day once a day in the morning ± food.

Side Effects: Common side effects are; abdominal pain, dyspnea, tachycardia, palpitation, headache, drowsiness.

* For action and nursing consideration refer to phenothiazines.

7. Quetiapine

Uses: Schizophrenia, bipolar mania.

Dosage: Adults (PO)

- Schizophrenia: Initially 25 mg 2 times/day can be increased slowly up to 300 mg/day in divided doses.
- Bipolar mania: 100 mg/day divided every 12 hours (Max: 400 mg/day).

Brands: 25, 50, 100, 200 mg Tab; Pincalm, Quel, Qutan.

Side Effects: Common side effects are; weight gain, dizziness, EPS, hypotension, constipation, dry mouth. Serious side effect is NMS.

* For action and nursing considerations refer phenothiazines.

8. Risperidone

Actions: Acts by antagonizing dopamine and serotonin in the CNS.

Uses: Schizophrenia, bipolar mania.

Dosage:

- Schizophrenia: Adults (PO): 1 mg 2 times/day (Max: 4 mg/day)
  (IM): 25 mg every 2 weeks
  Children 13–17 years (PO): 0.5 mg once a day (Max: 3 mg/day)
- Bipolar mania: Adults (PO): 2 mg/day once a day
  Children 13–17 years (PO): 0.5 mg once a day (Max: 2.5 mg/day).

Brands: 1, 2, 3, 4 mg Tab; Respidon, Sizodon, Speridon.

Side Effects: Common side effects are; constipation, dry mouth, diarrhea, weight gain, decrease libido, EPS, dizziness, insomnia, visual disturbances, cough, Serious side effect is neuroleptic malignant syndrome (NMS).

9. Ziprasidone

Action: Antagonism of dopamine type 2 and serotonin type 2 receptors.

Uses: Schizophrenia, bipolar mania.

Dosage: Adults.

- PO: Schizophrenia: 20 mg 2 times/day (Max: 80 mg 2 times/day)
  Mania: 40 mg day 1, 60 mg 2 times/day day 2 and 80 mg 2 times/day third day onwards
- IM: 10–20 mg day in divided doses (Max: 40 mg/day).

Brands: 20, 40, 60, 80 mg Cap; Zipsydon.

* For nursing consideration refer to phenothiazines.

Chapter 24

Antiretrovirals

Includes: (A) Non-nucleoside reverse transcriptase inhibitors
(B) Nucleoside reverse transcriptase inhibitors
(C) Protease inhibitors

General Nursing Considerations

- **Assess:** CBC, LFT, RFT, CD4 count, viral load, triglycerides, lipase, amylase, hepatitis 'B' and 'C' status. Change in signs and symptoms of HIV and secondary infection. Assess for rash specially in pediatric patients. Assess for CNS and psychiatric symptoms, peripheral neuropathy, signs of pancreatitis and hyperglycemia
- **Advise:** Take exactly as directed and comply with therapy even after symptoms subsides. Antiretrovirals do not cure HIV or reduce the transmission through sexual contact, blood transfusion or sharing needles. Avoid sex without condom, do not donate blood and share needles. They may cause dizziness or drowsiness, so advise avoiding activities requiring mental alertness. Notify immediately for signs and symptoms of hepatitis (pale stools, fever, flu-like symptoms, nausea, yellow eyes) and hyperglycemia (increased thrust or hunger, weight loss, increased frequency of urination). HIV drugs may cause changes in body fat distribution (increase over upper back, neck, breast and trunk; loss from face, arms and legs). Avoid crowded places and person with known infections
- **Desired Outcome:** Decrease in viral load and increase in CD4 counts, decrease in AIDS progression and opportunistic infections, decrease in viral load and protection of liver by chronic hepatitis-B, as applicable to particular drug.

(A) NON-NUCLEOSIDE REVERSE TRANSCRIPTASE INHIBITORS

Includes: 1. Efavirenz 2. Nevirapine

Action: Inhibits viral reverse transcriptase resulting in disruption of DNA synthesis and viral growth.

Use: HIV infection (in combination with one or more antiretroviral agents).

Side Effects: Common side effects are; nausea, vomiting, fever, anorexia, headache. Serious side effects are; hypersensitivity, SJS, hepatitis, rash.

1. Efavirenz

Dosage: PO ± food.

- Adults and children > 40 kg: 600 mg once daily
- Children 32.5–40 kg: 400 mg once a day, 25–32.5 kg: 350 mg once a day, 20–25 kg: 300 mg once a day, 15–20 kg: 250 mg once a day, 10–15 kg: 200 mg once a day.

Brands: 200 and 600 mg Tab; Efcure. 200 and 600 mg Cap; Estiva.

Nursing Consideration: Avoid it with high fat diet. Rash is usually seen within first 2 weeks. CNS and psychiatric symptoms are seen during 1st and 2nd day of therapy, to minimize these effects give drug at bedtime.

2. Nevirapine

Dosage: PO ± food.

- Adults: 200 mg once a day for 14 days then 200 mg BD
- Children >8 years: 4 mg/kg once a day for 14 days then 4 mg/kg BD
- Children 2 months – 8 years: 4 mg/kg once a day for 14 days then 7 mg/kg BD.

Brands: 200 mg Tab; 50 mg/5 mL Syp; Nevimune, Nevir.

(B) NUCLEOSIDE REVERSE TRANSCRIPTASE INHIBITORS

Includes:

1. Abacavir
2. Didanosine
3. Lamivudine
4. Stavudine
5. Tenofovir
6. Zidovudine

Action: Inhibits HIV reverse transcriptase causing disruption of DNA synthesis and viral growth.

Uses: HIV infection (in combination with one or more antiretrovirals). Lamivudine is also used for treatment of chronic hepatitis-B infection. Zidovudine in addition for chemoprophylaxis to reduce perinatal HIV transmission.

Side Effects: Common side effects are; nausea, vomiting, fever, rash anorexia, bone marrow suppression, peripheral neuropathy. Serious side effects include; hepatotoxicity, lactic acidosis, hypersensitivity, pancreatitis, seizures.

1. Abacavir

Dosage: PO ± food.

- Adults: 300 mg/dose 2 times/day
- Children >3 months: 8 mg/kg/dose 2 times/day (Max: 300 mg 2 times/day).

Brands: 300 mg Tab; Abavir, Abec.

Nursing Consideration: Stop drug at the first sign of hypersensitivity reaction.

2. Didanosine

Dosage: PO on empty stomach 30 minutes before or 2 hours after meal

- Adults: 125–200 mg/dose BD
- Children: 180–240 mg/m^2/day divided every 12 hours.

Brands: 250, 400 mg Tab; DD retro. 250 and 400 mg Cap; Virosine - DR.

3. Lamivudine

Dosage: PO ± Food.

- HIV infection:
  Adults and children > 12 years and ≥ 50 kg: 150 mg/dose 2 times/day.
  Children 3 month-12 years: 4 mg/kg/dose 2 times/day (Max: 150 mg/day BD).
- Chronic hepatitis-B:
  Adults: 100 mg once a day
  Children 2–17 years: 3 mg/kg/dose once a day.

Brands: 100 and 150 mg Tab; 50 mg/5 ml syp; Lamivir.

4. Stavudine

Dosage: PO ± food.

- Adults ≥ 60 kg: 40 mg/dose 2 times/day. Adults < 60 kg: 30 mg/dose 2 times/day
- Children > 1 month and < 30 kg: 1 mg/kg/dose 2 times/day.

Brands: 30 and 40 mg Tab; Virostav. 30 and 40 mg Cap; Stadine.

5. Tenofovir

Dosage: PO with meals. Adults: 300 mg once a day

Brands: 300 mg Tab; Tavin, Tenof

Nursing Consideration: It may cause hyperglycemia.

6. Zidovudine

Dosage: PO+food.

- HIV infection:
  Adults and children > 13 years: 200 mg/dose 3 times/day or 300 mg/dose 2 times/day
  Children 3 months–12 years: 90–180 mg/m^2 every 6 hours
- Chemoprophylaxis:
  Adults > 14 weeks pregnant: 100 mg 5 times/day until onset of labor
  Infants: 2 mg/kg/dose every 6 hours. Start within 12 hours of birth and give for 6 weeks.

Brands: 100 and 300 mg Tab; ZVD. 100 mg Cap; Retrovir. 50 mg/5 ml Syp; Zidovir.

Nursing Consideration: Patient should be in upright position while taking drug to minimize the risk of esophageal ulceration.

(C) PROTEASE INHIBITORS

Includes:

1. Atazanavir
2. Indinavir
3. Lopinavir
4. Nelfinavir
5. Ritonavir
6. Saquinavir

Action: Inhibits viral protease resulting in the formation of immature, noninfectious viral particles.

Uses: HIV infection in combination with other antiretrovirals.

Side Effects: Common side effects are; nausea, vomiting, rash, hyperglycemia, hyperlipidemia, diarrhea. Serious ones include; hypersensitivity, SJS, seizures, ketoacidosis.

1. Atazanavir

Dosage: PO + food to increase absorption.

Adults: 400 mg once a day.

Brands: 300 mg Tab; Reyataz

Nursing Consideration: May cause ECG changes.

2. Indinavir

Dosage: PO with water within 1 hour before or 2 hours after meal.

Adults: 800 mg/dose 3 times/day.

Brands: 400 mg Cap; Indivir, Virodin.

Nursing Consideration: Maintain adequate hydration to minimize the risk of nephrolithiasis.

3. Lopinavir

Dosage: PO + food to enhance absorption.

- Adults and children > 40 kg: 400 mg 2 times/day or 800 mg once a day
- Children 15–40 kg: 10 mg/kg/dose 2 times/day 7–15 kg: 13 mg/kg/dose 2 times/day.

Brands: Available in combination. Lopinavir 133.3 mg + Ritonavir 33.3 mg Tab and Cap; Lapimune, V-Letra.

Nursing Consideration: May cause hyperglycemia and ketoacidosis.

4. Nelfinavir

Dosage: PO+food.

- Adults and children > 13 years: 750 mg/dose 3 times/day
- Children 2–13 years: 20–30 mg/kg/dose 3 times/day.

Brands: 250 mg Tab; Nel, Nelvir.

5. Ritonavir

Dosage: PO + food.

- Adults: 600 mg/dose 2 times/day
- Children: 250 mg/m^2/dose 2 times/day.

Brands: 100 mg Cap; Ritovir, Ritomune.

Nursing Consideration: Can be combined with antiemetic and started at lower doses if nausea/vomiting occurs. May cause hyperglycemia and ketoacidosis.

6. Saquinavir

Dosage: PO within 2 hours of a meal to increase effectiveness.

Adults: 600 mg/dose 3 times/day.

Brands: 200 mg Cap; Saquin.

Nursing Consideration: Avoid exposure to sunlight and artificial light sources.

Chapter

25 Antithyroid Drugs

Include: 1. Carbimazole 2. Propylthiouracil

Action: Decreases synthesis of thyroid hormones.

Uses: Treatment of hyperthyroidism, also used during thyrotoxic crisis.

Nursing Consideration: Assess thyroid function test, CBC, LFT, PT, daily weight, signs and symptoms of hyperthyroidism or development of signs and symptoms of hypothyroidism. Monitor growth in children. It takes 6–12 weeks for the drug to produce full effect.

1. Carbimazole

Dosage: PO

- Adults: Initially 20–60 mg/day once or in divided doses. Maintenance dose is 5–15 mg/day for at least 1 year
- Children: 4–12 years: Initially 15 mg/day, titrate further doses.

Brands: 5, 10, 20 mg Tab; Neomercazole, Thyrocab.

Side Effects: Sore throat, fever, oral ulcer, leukopenia, headache, hypothyroidism.

2. Propylthiouracil

Dosage: PO with meal.

- Adults: Initially 300–900 mg/day once or in divided doses. Maintenance dose is 50–600 mg/day in divided doses
- Children >10 years: 50–300 mg/day in divided doses. 6–10 years: 50–150 mg/day in divided doses.

Brands: 50 mg Tab; PTU.

Side Effects: Common side effects are; nausea, vomiting, diarrhea, hepatitis, rash, decreased taste, cervical lymphadenopathy. Serious one is agranulocytosis.

Nursing Consideration: Stop therapy if cervical lymphadenopathy or rash appears.

Chapter

26 Antituberculars

Include: 1. Cycloserine
2. Ethambutol
3. Ethionamide
4. Isoniazid
5. Pyrazinamide
6. Rifampicin
7. Streptomycin

General Nursing Considerations

- **Assess:** CBC, LFT, RFT, input and output, mycobacterial study and susceptibility test, lung sounds, characteristics of sputum, mental status
- **Administration:** Give along with antiemetic if vomiting occur
- **Advise:** Comply with dosage and duration even after symptoms have subsided. Avoid alcohol use
- **Desired Outcome:** Resolution of signs and symptoms of tuberculosis (fever, cough, sputum, weight gain, increased appetite, etc.), improvement in chest X-ray, decrease in acid fast bacteria in sputum samples.

1. Cycloserine

Action: Inhibits bacterial cell wall synthesis.

Uses: Adjunct in treatment of pulmonary and extrapulmonary tuberculosis, acute UTI caused by *E. coli* or enterobacter species.

Dosage: PO ± food.

- TB: Adults: 250 mg 2 times/day for 14 days then 500 mg–1 g/day in 2 divided doses. Children: 10–20 mg/kg/day divided every 12 hours
- UTI: Adults: 250 mg 2 times/day for 14 days.

Brands: 250 mg Cap; Cyclorine, Myser.

Side Effects: Megaloblastic anemia, convulsions, CHF.

Nursing Consideration: Avoid activities requiring alertness. Exposure to sunlight and artificial light sources should be avoided. Some of the neurotoxic effects may be prevented by concomitant use of pyridoxine. Sedatives may be effective in reducing tremors or anxiety. Supplement vitamin B_{12} and folic acid during therapy.

2. Ethambutol

Action: Inhibits growth of mycobacteria.

Uses: Treatment of active tuberculosis.

Dosage: PO + food.

Adults and Children: 15–25 mg/kg/day once daily (Max: 2.5 g/day).

Brands: 200, 400, 600, 800 mg Tab; Combutal, Zytham.

Side Effects: Common side effects are; optic neuritis, headache, abdominal pain, GI upset. Serious side effects include; hepatitis, thrombocytopenia.

Nursing Consideration: Assess visual function frequently and avoid use in children whose visual acuity cannot be determined and monitored.

3. Ethionamide

Action: Inhibits peptide synthesis.

Uses: Treatment of tuberculosis.

Dosage: PO + food.

- Adults: 500–1000 mg/day in 3 divided doses
- Children: 15–20 mg/kg/day in 3 divided doses (Max: 1 g/day)

Brands: 250 mg Tab; Enamide, Ethide.

Side Effects: Anorexia, nausea, vomiting, convulsions, thrombocytopenia.

Nursing Consideration: If used along with cycloserine and isoniazid chances of nervous system adverse effects are increased. Supplement pyridoxine to prevent neurotoxic effects. Do periodic ophthalmological examination.

4. Isoniazid

Action: Inhibits cell wall synthesis.

Uses: Treatment and prevention of tuberculosis.

Dosage: PO, given 1 hour before or 2 hours after meal with water.

- Treatment: Adults; 5–10 mg/kg/day (usual dose: 300 mg)
  Infants and children; 10–15 mg/kg/day once daily (Max: 300 mg/day)
- Prophylaxis: Adults; 300 mg/day
  Infants and children; 10 mg/kg/day once daily (Max: 300 mg/day).

Brands: 100 mg Tab; Isonex. 300 mg Tab; Isonex forte.

Side Effects: Common side effect is peripheral neuropathy. Serious side effects ones include; drug induced hepatitis, convulsions, encephalopathy, thrombocytopenia.

Nursing Consideration: Overdoses are treated with pyridoxine and may be used concurrently to prevent neuropathy.

5. Pyrazinamide

Action: Bacteriostatic agent.

Use: Treatment of active tuberculosis.

Dosage: PO

Adults, children and infants: 15–30 mg/kg/day in divided doses (Max: 2 g/day).

Brands: 250, 500, 750 mg Tab; Piraldina, PZA-CIBA.

Side Effects: Common side effects are; GI upset, arthralgia, myalgia, hyperuricemia. Serious side effects are; hepatotoxicity, hemolytic anemia.

Nursing Consideration: Increase fluid intake (2–3 L/day). Monitor uric acid level. Avoid exposure to sun and artificial light. Combination therapy with isoniazid may cause fatal and severe hepatotoxic reactions.

6. Rifampicin

Action: Inhibits RNA synthesis.

Uses: Treatment of active tuberculosis. Elimination of meningococci from a symptomatic carriers, prophylaxis in contacts of patient with *H. influenzae* type-B infection.

Dosage: Give PO on empty stomach 1 hour before or 2 hours after meal with water.

- TB: Adults: 10 mg/kg/day once daily (Max: 600 mg/day)
  Infants and children: 10–20 mg/kg/day divided every 12 hours
- Meningococcal prophylaxis: Give for 2 days
  Adults: 600 mg every 12 hours
  Infants and children: 20 mg/kg/day divided every 12 hours
  < 1 month: 10 mg/kg/day divided every 12 hours
- *H. influenzae* prophylaxis: Give for 4 days
  Adults: 600 mg/day once a day
  Infants and children: 20 mg/kg/day once a day
  Neonates: 10 mg/kg/day once a day.

Brands: 300, 450 and 600 mg Tab; Zucox. 300, 450, 600 mg. Cap; R-cin. 100 mg/5 ml Syp; R-cin.

Side Effects: Common side effects are; abdominal pain, diarrhea, nausea, vomiting, heartburn, red discoloration of body fluids. Serious side effects are; hematuria, leukopenia, pancreatitis.

7. Streptomycin

Action: Inhibit protein synthesis in bacterial cell wall.

Uses: Treatment of active tuberculosis, enterococcal endocarditis, plague.

Dosage: IM

- Adults: TB: 20–40 mg/kg/day (Max: 1 g/day)
  Plague: 2 g/day in divided doses until patient is afebrile for at least 3 days
  Endocarditis: 1 g every 12 hours for 2 weeks, then 500 mg every 12 hours for 4 weeks along with penicillin
- Children: TB: 20–40 mg/kg/day once daily
  Other infections: 20–30 mg/kg/day divided every 12 hours.

Brands: 750 and 1000 mg vial; Ambistryn, ISOS.

Nursing Consideration: Store in refrigerator. Give deep IM, maximum concentration allowed is 500 mg/mL.

For side effects and nursing consideration refer Antibiotics—aminoglycosides (Chapter 7, Page no. 40).

Chapter

27 Antitussives/ Expectorants

Include: Antitussives and expectorants.

Antitussives act by suppressing the cough reflex and should only be used for dry unproductive cough or if cough is tiring, disturbing sleep or is hazardous (cardiac diseases, piles, ocular surgery, hernia). Expectorants act by liquefying and reducing viscosity of thick tenacious secretions, facilitating its removal by cough.

General Nursing Considerations

- **Assess:** Respiratory rate, rhythm, distress, lung sounds, frequency and type of cough, amount and type of secretions
- **Administration:** Avoid in acute attack of asthma or severe bronchospasm. Do mechanical suction if cough is insufficient to remove excess bronchial secretions. Unless contraindicated, maintain fluid intake of 1500–2000 mL/day to decrease viscosity of secretions
- **Advise:** Sit upright and take several breath before attempting cough; turn frequently, limit talking, stop smoking. Maintain good moisture in the environmental air, avoid fumes, dust and perfumes, and advise taking frequent sips of water to decrease frequency of dry cough
- **Desired Outcome:** Decrease in cough and distress.

1. Acetylcysteine

Action: Opens disulfide bonds in mucoproteins present in sputum, increases hepatic glutathione required in acetaminophen overdoses.

Uses: As mucolytic in cough, acetaminophen toxicity.

Dosage: Priming with aerosolized bronchodilator 10–15 minutes prior to therapy is beneficial.

- Nebulization: Infants: 1–2 mL of 20% solution 3–4 times/day
  Children: 3–5 mL of 20% solution 3–4 times/day
  Adults: 5–10 mL of 20% solution 3–4 times/day
- Intratracheal: Adults and children: 1–2 mL of 10–20% solution every 1–4 hours as needed
- Acetaminophen toxicity: Begin within 8 hours of ingestion
  PO: Initially 140 mg/kg followed by 17 doses of 70 mg/kg every 4 hours

IV: Initially 150 mg/kg over 15 minutes followed by 4 hourly infusion of 50 mg/kg, followed by a 16 hour infusion of 100 mg/kg.

Brands: 200 mg/mL Inj; Mucomix.

Side Effects: Common side effects are; dizziness, drowsiness, nausea, rhinorrhea. Serious side effects are; bronchospasm, hemoptysis, hepatotoxicity.

Nursing Considerations

- **Assess:** Antidotal use, LFT, PT, serum urea, blood glucose, serum electrolyte
- **Administration:** Dilute first IV dose in 250 mL of D5W, second in 500 mL and third in 1000 mL of D5W. Give PO 1 hour before meal for better absorption. Use within 96 hours of opening and store in refrigerator. Suction machine should be ready before intratracheal use
- **Advise:** Avoid activities requiring alertness and other CNS depressants. Unpleasant odor decreases with repeated use
- **Desired Outcome:** Decrease in cough and secretions, absence of hepatic damage.

2. Ambroxol

Action: Alters secretion and physical properties of mucus facilitating its removal.

Use: As mucolytic in cough.

Dosage: PO

- Adults: 60–120 mg/day divided every 8 hourly
- Children: < 2 years, 7.5 mg 2 times/day. 2–5 years, 7.5 mg 3 times/day. 6–12 years, 15 mg 2 or 3 times/day.

Brands: 30 mg Tab; Ambrodil, Ambrolite. 30 mg/5 mL Syp; Ambrodil, Mucolite. Also available in combinations.

Side Effects: Rhinorrhea, lacrimation, GI discomfort.

3. Ammonium Chloride

Action: Lowers urinary pH, correction of alkalosis.

Uses: Metabolic alkalosis, expectorant, systemic and urinary acidifier.

Dosage:

- Alkalosis: Adults and children: IV infusion of 0.9–1.3 mL/min of 2.14% solution
- Acidifier: Adults (PO): 4–12 g/day in divided doses. Children (PO): 75 mg/kg/day in divided doses
- Expectorant: Adults (PO): 250–500 mg every 4 hours. Children (PO): 125–250 mg every 4 hours.

Brands: Ammonium chloride 100 mg + Diphenhydramine 10 mg + Codeine 10 mg + Ephedrine 7 mg per 5 mL; Bronolax.

Side Effects: GI discomfort, nausea, vomiting, twitching, hyperreflexia, hypokalemia, apnea.

Nursing Considerations

- **Assess:** LFT, serum electrolytes and SPO_2, serum chloride; input and output
- **Administration:** Per oral with meals
- **Advise:** Increase potassium in diet (banana, oranges, spinach, dry fruits)
- **Desired Outcome:** Decrease in alkalosis, increase urinary acidosis, productive cough.

4. Bromhexine

Dosage: PO. Adults: 8 mg 3 times/day. Children (5–10 years): 4 mg 3 times/day, (1–5 years): 4 mg 2 times/day.

Brands: 8 mg Tab; 4 mg/5 mL liquid, Bisolvon, Bromhexine. Also available in various combinations.

- For action, uses and side effects refer to ambroxol.

5. Carbocisteine

Action: As acetylcysteine.

Uses: As mucolytic in cough.

Dosage: PO. Adults: 250–750 mg 3 times/day. Children: 125–250 mg 3 times/day.

Brands: 100, 375 mg Cap; 250 mg/5 mL Syp; Mucodyne. Also available in combinations.

6. Codeine

For details refer to analgesics—narcotics (Chapter 1, Page no. 9).

7. Dextromethorphan

Action: Acts in the cough center in the medulla.

Uses: As antitussive in nonproductive cough.

Dosage: PO

- Adults and Childern > 12 years: 30 mg every 6–8 hours (Max: 120 mg/day)
- Children 6–12 years: 15 mg every 6–8 hours (Max: 60 mg/day)
- Children 2–6 years: 2.5–7.5 mg every 6–8 hours (Max: 30 mg/day).

Brands: 30 mg/5 mL Syp; Lastuss-LA. 10 mg Tab; Lastuss-CT. Available in combination with cetirizine, ambroxol, chlorpheniramine, phenylpropanolamine, etc.

Side Effects: Nausea, high doses may cause dizziness and sedation.

Nursing Consideration: Do not give fluid immediately after per oral dose to prevent drug dilution.

8. Diphenhydramine

Action: Antihistaminic at H_1 receptor sites, CNS depressant and anticholinergic.

Uses: Relief of allergic symptoms, prevention of motion sickness, antitussive, dystonic reaction.

Dosage: PO + food.

- Phenothiazine induced dystonic and moderate to severe allergic reaction:
  Adults: 25–50 mg every 4 hours (Max: 400 mg/day)
  Children: 5 mg/kg/day divided every 8 hours (Max: 300 mg/day)
- Mild allergic rhinitis and motion sickness:
  Adults and children ≥ 2 years: 25–40 mg every 4–6 hours
  Children 6 to < 12 years: 12.5–25 mg every 4–6 hours
  Children 2 to ≤ 6 years: 6.25 mg every 4-6 hours
- Antitussive:
  Adults and children ≤ 12 years: 12 mg every 4 hours (Max: 150 mg/day)
  Children 6 to < 12 years: 12.5 mg every 4 hours (Max: 75 mg/day)
  Children 2 to ≤ 6 years: 6.25 mg every 4 hours (Max: 37.5 mg/day).

Brands: 25 mg Cap; 12.5 mg/5 mL syp; 2 to ≤ 6 years. Benadryl. Also available in various combinations.

Side Effects: Dry mouth, anorexia, drowsiness, paradoxical excitation.

Nursing Considerations

- **Assess:** Urticaria, nasal stuffiness, rhinorrhea, nausea, vomiting, itching, rash
- **Administration:** When using for motion sickness, administer at least 1–2 hours before journey
- **Desired Outcome:** Control in dystonic reactions, motion sickness and cough.

9. Guaifensin

Action: Decreases viscosity of mucus by increasing respiratory tract fluid.

Uses: As expectorant in cough.

Dosage: PO

- Adults and children ≥ 12 years: 200–400 mg every 4 hours
- Children 6 to < 12 years: 100–200 mg every 4 hours
- Children 2 to < 6 years: 50–100 mg every 4 hours.

Brands: Available in various combinations with dextromethorphan, chlorpheniramine, codeine, etc.

Side Effects: GI discomfort, rashes, headache, dizziness.

Nursing Consideration: Each dose should be given with large quantity of water to ensure proper action.

Chapter

28 Antiulcers

Include: (A) Antacids (B) H_2 Antagonists (C) Proton Pump Inhibitors (D) Miscellaneous

(A) ANTIULCER—ANTACIDS

Include:
1. Aluminium Hydroxide
2. Calcium Carbonate
3. Magaldrate
4. Magnesium Hydroxide
5. Magnesium Trisilicate
6. Sodium Bicarbonate

Action: These are basic substances which neutralize gastric acid.

Uses: Duodenal and gastric ulcers, gastric hypersecretory conditions, GERD, prevention of GI bleeding in ill patients.

Side Effects: Aluminium salts causes constipation, hypophosphatemia. Calcium salts causes hypercalcemia, hypophosphatemia, constipation, diarrhea, belching, flatulence, abdominal distension. Magnesium salts causes GI upset, diarrhea, hypermagnesemia. Sodium salts causes alkalosis, electrolyte imbalance.

General Nursing Considerations

- **Assess:** Input and output, urinary retention, dysuria. Abdominal or epigastric pain, frank or occult blood, emesis, gastric aspirate
- **Administration:** Aluminium and magnesium salts are combined to balance the side effects. Use with caution in patients of renal disease or dehydration. All products should be given with 200 mL of water to ensure good absorption in stomach. Change antacid if side effects occurs. Administer 1–3 hours after meals and at bedtime for maximum effects. Antacids causes premature dissolution and absorption of EC tablets so give at a gap of 1 hour. Do not allow oral medicine within 1–2 hours of antacid use
- **Advise:** Chew tablet thoroughly before swallowing and shake suspensions well before use. To avoid constipation use bulk food, plenty of fluids and laxatives. Stop smoking, alcohol, spices
- **Desired Outcome:** Decrease in abdominal pain, emesis, distension, bleeding, symptoms of GERD.

Dosage: PO (Various salts).

- Aluminium hydroxide and magnesium hydroxide combinations:
  Infants: 1-2 mL/kg/dose after meals and at bedtime
  Children: 5-15 mL every 3-6 hours after meals and at bedtime
  Adults: 15-45 mL every 3-6 hours after meals and at bedtime
- Sodium bicarbonate: Adults and Children > 6 years: 1-5 mg/dose every 4-6 hours
- Magaldrate: 500-1000 mg twice to thrice daily
- Calcium carbonate: 2-5 years; 500 mg as needed. 6-11 years; 800 mg as needed. > 11 years and adults; 1000-3000 mg as needed
- Magnesium trisilicate: 100-500 mg 3 times/day.

Brands:

- Digene susp: Mag hyd. 185 mg + Alum hyd. 830 mg+Simethicon 50 mg/10 mL
- Digene tab: Mag. hyd. 25 mg + Alum. hyd. 300 mg + Mg. Silicate 50 mg
- Gelusil liquid: Alum hyd. 300 mg + Mag. hyd. 150 mg + Dimethicon 125 mg/ 5 mL
- Gelusil Tab: Alum hyd. 300 mg + Mag. hyd. 150 mg + Dimethicon 125 mg + Mag. Silicate 75 mg.

(B) ANTIULCER—H_2 ANTAGONISTS

Include: 1. Cimetidine 2. Famotidine 3. Ranitidine

Action: Acts by blocking histamine induced gastric secretions

Uses: Duodenal and gastric ulcers, gastric hypersecretory conditions, GERD, prevention of GI bleeding in ill patients.

Side Effects: Common side effects are; headache, diarrhea, confusion. Serious side effects are; neutropenia, thrombocytopenia, exfoliative dermatitis.

General Nursing Considerations

- **Assess:** BP, HR, input and output specially during IV use, CBC. Elderly for confusion. Abdominal or epigastric pain, frank or occult blood, emesis, gastric aspirate
- **Administration:** Give with meal for prolonged drug effect. Give IV slowly as rapid administration may cause hypotension and arrhythmias. Avoid antacids for 1 hour and sucralfate for 2 hours if used concurrently. If using once daily give at bedtime to enhance effect. PO ± food. Dosage may need to decrease in impaired renal function
- **Advise:** Gynecomastia and impotence if occurs are reversible. May cause false positive urine protein test. Avoid smoking, alcohol, coffee, spices, NSAIDs to enhance effect
- **Desired Outcome:** Decrease in abdominal pain, distension, emesis, bleeding, symptoms of GERD.

1. Cimetidine

Dosage: PO

- Adults: Active ulcer: 200 mg 4 times/day or 800 mg at bedtime. GERD: 800 mg 2 times/day or 400 mg 4 times/day. Hypersecretory conditions: 300–600 mg every 6 hours
- Children: 20–40 mg/kg/day divided every 6 hours.

Brands: 200, 400 mg Tabs; Cimetiget, Ulciban.

2. Famotidine

Dosage: PO, IV

- Adults and children > 12 years: Peptic ulcer: 20 mg/day at bedtime for 4–8 weeks
  GERD: 20 mg 2 times/day for 6 weeks
- Ped 1–12 years: Peptic ulcer: 0.5 mg/kg/day divided every 12 hours.
  GERD: 1 mg/kg/day divided every 12 hours.

Nursing Consideration: For IV use dilute in NS/D5W/RL in a concentration of 4 mg/mL and give at a rate of 10 mg/min.

Brands: 20, 40 mg Tabs; 10 mg/mL Inj; Famocid, Famonite.

3. Ranitidine

Dosage:

- Adults and Children >16 years:
  Gastric and duodenal ulcer, GERD: PO: 150 mg/dose 2 times/day or 300 mg at bedtime
  Hypersecretory conditions: PO: 150 mg BD. IV: 50 mg/dose every 6–8 hours
- Children 1 month–16 years:
  Gastric and duodenal ulcer, GERD: PO, IV: 2–4 mg/kg/day divided every 8–12 hours.

Brands: 150, 300 mg Tabs; 25 mg/mL Inj; Aciloc, Histac, Rantac.

Nursing Consideration: For IV dilute in NS/RL/D5W in a concentration of 2.5 mg/mL and give at the rate of 10 mg/min.

(C) ANTIULCER—PROTON PUMP INHIBITORS

Include:
1. Esomeprazole
2. Lansoprazole
3. Omeprazole
4. Pantoprazole
5. Rabeprazole

Action: Acts by inhibiting proton pumps, thereby decreasing gastric acid secretion.

Uses: Duodenal and gastric ulcers, gastric hypersecretory conditions, GERD, prevention of GI bleeding in ill patients.

Side Effects: Dizziness, headache, diarrhea, abdominal pain, dry mouth, fatigue.

General Nursing Considerations

- **Assess:** Abdominal or epigastric pain, frank or occult blood loss, emesis, gastric aspirate. Monitor vitals before and during IV use
- **Administration:** Take before meals, preferably in the morning. Give antacids 1 hour prior and H_2 antagonists 1 hour later if used concurrently. If given via NG tube mix with sterile water or sodium bicarbonate. Use for short period of time as these drugs decrease total gastric secretion
- **Advise:** To increase the effect avoid alcohol, smoking, NSAIDs, spices. Hypoglycemia may occur in diabetic patients
- **Desired Outcome:** Decrease in abdominal pain, distension, emesis, bleeding, symptoms of GERD.

1. Esomeprazole

Dosage:
- Adults: (PO): 20–40 mg once or twice daily. (IV): 20 mg once daily
- Children 12–17 years: (PO): 20 mg once daily.

Brands: 20, 40 mg Tabs; Esoz, Nuloc. 40 mg Inj; Esoz, Nexpro.

Nursing Consideration: For IV use dilute 1 vial in NS /RL/D_5W and administer over 3 minutes. Absorption is decreased upto 50% if taken along with food.

2. Lansoprazole

Dosage:
- Adults and children ≥ 12 years: PO: Duodenal ulcer: 15 mg once daily. Gastric ulcer: 30 mg once daily. GERD: 15 mg once daily
- Children < 12 years: 0.5–1.6 mg/kg once daily or in divided doses.

Brands: 15, 30 mg Tabs; Acilanz. 15, 30 mg cap; Lansofast, Lanzol.

3. Omeprazole

Dosage: PO
- Adults and adolescents: Duodenal ulcer/GERD/Heart burn: 20 mg/day. Gastric ulcer: 40 mg/day
- Children: Ulcers, esophagitis, GERD: 1 mg/kg/day once or twice daily.

Brands: 20 mg Tab; Omcid, Omegold, 20, 40 mg Cap; Ocid, Omez.

4. Pantoprazole

Dosage:
- Adults: GERD (PO): 40 mg once. (IV): 40 mg once daily. Gastric hypersecretory conditions (PO): 40 mg twice daily. (IV): 80 mg every 12 hours
- Children: 0.5–1 mg/kg/day.

Brands: 20, 40 mg Tabs; Aciban, Pan. 40 mg Inj; Apanta, Pansa.

Nursing Consideration: For IV dilute powder in 10 mL NS, further dilute in NS/D_5W/RL to a final concentration of 0.4–0.8 mg/mL, then infuse at the rate of 5 mL/min. Patient on IV should be shifted to oral as soon as possible.

5. Rabeprazole

Dosage: Adults: GERD, ulcer, esophagitis: 20 mg once or twice daily.

Brands: 10, 20 mg Tabs; Rablet, Rapeed, Repraz.

(D) ANTIULCER—MISCELLANEOUS

Sucralfate

Action: Forms physical barrier of ulcer adherent complex that protects it against gastric acid, pepsin and bile acids.

Uses: Duodenal and gastric ulcers, gastric hypersecretory conditions, GERD, prevention of GI bleeding in ill patients.

Dosage: PO

- Adults: Ulcer prophylaxis: 1 g every 12 hours
- Duodenal ulcer, gastric ulcer, GERD: 1 g every 6 hours
- Children: 40–80 mg/kg/day divided every 6 hours.

Brands: 1 g Tab; 500 and 1000 mg/10 mL susp; Pepsigard, Sucral.

Side Effects: Causes constipation, drowsiness, indigestion, dry mouth.

Nursing Consideration:

- **Assess:** Abdominal or epigastric pain, frank or occult blood, emesis, gastric aspirate. Input and output, HR, BP specially in renal patients due to accumulation of aluminium
- **Administration:** Give empty stomach 1 hour before meal and at bedtime. If antacids used concurrently administer 30 minutes before or after sucralfate dosage
- **Advise:** Don't crush or chew tablet, shake suspension well before use. Interferes with adsorption of Vitamin A, D, E and K; supplement them on long-term use. Avoid smoking, alcohol, spices, NSAIDs. They may cause constipation; so increase in fiber and fluid intake and do regular exercise should be advised
- **Desired Outcome:** Decrease in abdominal pain, distension, emesis, bleed, symptoms of GERD.

Chapter

29 Antivirals

Include:

1. Acyclovir
2. Amantadine
3. Famciclovir
4. Ganciclovir
5. Lamivudine
6. Ribavarin
7. Valacyclovir

Action: Interferes with DNA synthesis that is needed for viral replication.

Side Effects: Common side effects are; nausea, vomiting, diarrhea, headache, vaginitis, moniliasis, phlebitis. Serious side effects are; fatal metabolic encephalopathy, acute renal failure, blood dyscrasias.

General Nursing Considerations

- **Assess:** CBC, LFT, RFT, culture and sensitivity, signs and symptoms of anemia, bowel pattern, skin lesions, bleeding (internal/external), eye lesions, monitor neurologic status in herpes encephalitis patients, postherpetic neuralgia
- **Administration:** Increase fluid intake to 3 L/day to decrease crystalluria during IV therapy. Give it round the clock to maintain optimal drug level. Rotate infusion site to prevent phlebitis
- **Advise:** Drugs do not cure, but they only control symptoms. Even after symptoms subsides drugs should be taken for full course of therapy. Take precautions to prevent spread of virus as the drug do not prevent transmission. Report superinfection (fever, sore throat, fatigue, etc.). Partners of genital herpes must use condoms to prevent reinfection and avoid sex while lesions are present. Loose clothing should be worn to prevent lesion irritation
- **Desired Outcome:** Absence or control of signs and symptoms of viral infection. Crusting and healing of lesions. Healing and decrease of pain in herpes zoster. Decrease in intensity of chickenpox. Decrease in frequency of recurrences.

1. Acyclovir

Uses: Treatment of initial disease and prophylaxis of recurrent mucosal and cutaneous herpes simplex (HSV-1 and 2) infections, herpes simplex encephalitis, herpes zoster infection, varicella zoster infection.

Dosage:
- Genital HSV, first episode: Adults and children (PO): 400 mg every 4 hours for 7–10 days. (Maximum dose in children is 80 mg/kg/day in 5 divided doses). (IV): 15 mg/kg/day divided every 8 hours for 5–7 days
- Recurrent genital HSV: Adults (PO): 800–1000 mg/day in 5 divided doses
- Herpes simplex encephalitis (IV): Adults and Children: 30 mg/kg/day divided every 8 hours for 14–21 days
- Herpes zoster in immunocompetent patients (PO): Adults: 4000 mg/day in 5 divided doses for 5–7 days
- Varicella zoster in immunocompetent host: Start within 24 hours of onset of rash. Adults and children (PO): 80 mg/kg/day in 4 divided doses for 5 days. (IV): 30 mg/kg/day in 4 divided doses for 7–10 days.

Brands: 200, 400, 800 mg Tab; Acivir, Ocuvir. 25 mg/mL Inj; Zovirax, Ovir.

Nursing Consideration: PO±food. Maintain good hydration specially during first 24 hours of IV therapy to prevent crystalluria. For IV use dilute in SWI in a concentration of 7 mg/mL and infuse over 1 hour as rapid rate may cause renal damage.

2. Amantadine

For details refer to antiparkinson agents (Chapter 21).

3. Famciclovir

Uses: Acute herpes zoster infection, treatment or suppression of recurrent herpes genitalis in immunocompetent patient.

Dosage: Adults: PO ± food.
- Herpes zoster: 500 mg every 8 hours for 7 days. Initiate within 48 hours of rash onset
- Recurrent genital herpes: 1000 mg twice for 1 day
- Suppression of recurrent genital herpes: 250 mg twice daily for upto 1 year.

Brands: 250 and 500 mg Tab; Famtrex, Virovir.

4. Ganciclovir

Uses: Treatment of CMV retinitis in immunocompromised patients and prevention of CMV disease in transplant patient.

Dosage: IV
- Retinitis: Adults and children > 3 months:
  Induction dose: 10 mg/kg/day divided every 12 hourly for 14–21 days
  Maintenance: 5 mg/kg/day as single dose for 5 days in a week
- Prevention dose: Adults and children: 10 mg/kg/day divided every 12 hours for 7–14 days, followed by 5 mg/kg/day once daily for 5 days in a week
- Maintenance following IV induction (PO):
  Adults: 100 mg, 3 times/day, children: 30 mg/kg/dose every 8 hours.

Brands: 250 mg Cap; 500 mg/Vial; Cytovene.

Nursing Consideration: Diagnosis of CMV retinitis should be confirmed by ophthalmoscopy. It should be given per oral with food. For IV dilute in 100 mL of NS/RL/D_5W in a maximum concentration of 10 mg/mL and infuse over 1 hour. Do regular ophthalmic examination every 6 weeks.

5. Lamivudine

For details refer—antiretrovirals (Chapter 24).

6. Ribavarin

Uses: Treatment of lower respiratory tract infection caused by RSV in infants and young children with compromising conditions (BPD, CHD, prematurity).

Dosage:

- Inhalation: Adults, children and infants: Dilute 6 mg of ribavirin in 300 mL of sterile water and nebulize for 12–18 hrs/day for 3–7 days as continuous inhalation. For intermittent inhalation give 33.3 mL over 2 hours 3 times/day for 3–7 days
- PO: Children: 10 mg/kg/day in divided doses.

Brands: 100 and 200 mg Cap; 50 mg/5 mL Syp; Ribavin, Virazide.

Nursing Consideration: PO+food. Assess sputum, respiratory and fluid status. Treatment for RSV infection should be given within 3 days. Patient may have blurred vision, dizziness and photosensitivity during therapy. Do inhalation in a well-ventilated room.

7. Valacyclovir

Uses: Treatment of herpes zoster, treatment or suppression of genital herpes.

Dosage: PO±food.

- Herpes zoster: Adults (PO): 1 g 3 times/day for 7 days
- Genital herpes: Adults (PO): Treatment of first episode 1 g 2 times/day for 10 days. Recurrences, 500 mg 2 times/day for 3 days.

Brands: 500 and 1000 mg Cap; Valcivir.

Nursing Consideration: Start therapy within 48 hours.

Chapter

30 Bone Resorption Inhibitors

Include: 1. Alendronate 2. Pamidronate 3. Raloxifene

Action:

- Alendronate and raloxifene inhibit bone resorption by inhibiting hydroxyapatite crystal dissolution and osteoclast activity
- Raloxifene binds to estrogen receptors in the bone and decreases bone resorption and bone turnover.

General Nursing Considerations

- **Assess:** BP, input and output, bone density before and during therapy, phosphorus, magnesium, potassium, calcium, alkaline phosphatase, serum electrolytes, RFT, skull size, headache, bone pain
- **Administration:** Should not be used in patients with hypocalcemia and vit. D deficiency. Correct hypocalcemia and vit-D deficiency before starting therapy
- **Advise:** Do regular exercise, calcium supplementation, stop smoking and alcohol
- **Desired Outcome:** Prevention and decrease in osteoporosis, decreased progression of Paget's disease, increased bone mass and prevention of fractures.

1. Alendronate

Uses: Prevention and treatment of osteoporosis in; postmenopausal women, men or due to corticosteroid therapy.

Dosage: Adults: PO:

- Treatment of osteoporosis: 10 mg once daily or 70 mg once weekly
- Prevention of osteoporosis: 5 mg once daily or 35 mg once weekly
- Treatment of corticosteroid induced osteoporosis: 5 mg once daily.

Brands: 5, 10, 35, 70 mg Tabs; Bifosa, Osteofos.

Side Effects: Headache, blurred vision, esophageal ulcers, acid regurgitation.

Nursing Consideration: Administer in the morning with a glass of water and let the patient remain upright for 30 minutes to 1 hour.

2. Pamidronate

Uses: Management of hypercalcemia of malignancy, multiple myeloma, Paget's disease.

Dosage: Adults: IV:

- Hypercalcemia of malignancy: 30–90 mg can be repeated >1 week
- Multiple myeloma: 90 mg monthly
- Paget's disease: 60–90 mg single dose.

Brands: 30, 60, 90 mg Inj: Bonapam, Pamidria.

Side Effects: Nausea, fever, pain, hypokalemia, hypocalcemia, hypophosphatemia.

Nursing Consideration: Maintain enough hydration PO or IV to maintain a urine output of 2 L per day. Dilute 1 vial in 10 mL of sterile water and this is further diluted to 500–1000 mL of NS and infused over 6–24 hours. Assess for seizure activity, incorporate seizure precautions. Avoid diet rich in calcium.

3. Raloxifene

Uses: Treatment and prevention of osteoporosis in postmenopausal women, reduction of risk of breast cancer in postmenopausal women with osteoporosis.

Dosage: Adults: PO: 60 mg once daily.

Brands: 60 mg Tabs; Bonmax, Ralofen.

Side Effects: Hot flushes, leg cramps, deep vein thrombosis, stroke.

Chapter

31 Cholinergics

Include: 1. Bethanechol 2. Neostigmine 3. Pyridostigmine

Action: Prevents the breakdown of acetylcholine so that its concentration is increased and thus has a prolonged effect. Bethanechol stimulates cholinergic receptors in the smooth muscle.

Side Effects: Serious side effects are; seizures, bronchospasm. Common side effects are; abdominal cramps, diarrhea, excess salivation, sweating, nausea, vomiting.

General Nursing Considerations

- **Assess:** PR, BP, respiration, urinary retention or incontinence, neuromuscular status (vital capacity, diplopia, chewing, ptosis, swallowing), overdose and underdose (muscle weakness, dysphagia, dyspnea), abdominal status (bowel sounds, distension), reversal effect of neuromuscular blockage
- **Administration:** When using as an antidote to nondepolarizing neuromuscular blocking agents, atropine should be used prior or concurrently for prevention and treatment of bradycardia. Use large doses after exercise or fatigue
- **Advise:** Take exactly as directed. Medicine is not a cure, it only relieves symptoms in myasthenia gravis. Myasthenia patient should keep gap between activities to avoid fatigue
- **Desired Outcome:** Increased muscle strength, hand grasp, improved gait, chewing, swallowing. Relief of postoperative nonobstructive urinary retention, reversal of effects of neuromuscular blocking agents as applicable to particular drug.

1. Bethanechol

Uses: Treatment of nonobstructive urinary retention and retention due to neurogenic bladder.

Dosage: PO, given empty stomach.

- Adults: 10–15 mg 4 times/day
- Children: 0.1–0.2 mg/kg/dose 3 times/day.

Brands: 25 mg Tab; Bethacol, Urotonin.

Nursing Consideration: Change position slowly to avoid orthostatic hypotension.

2. Neostigmine

Uses: Treatment of myasthenia gravis, reversal of nondepolarizing neuromuscular blocking agents.

Dosage:

- Myasthenia gravis:
  Adults (PO): Initially 15 mg every 3–4 hours, can be increased daily
  (IM, IV): 0.5–2.5 mg every 1–3 hours
  Children (PO): 2 mg/kg/day in divided doses
  (IM, IV): 0.01–0.04 mg/kg every 2–4 hours
- Reversal of nondepolarizing neuromuscular blockade (IV):
  Adults: 0.5–0.25 mg (Max dose: 5 mg)
  Children: 0.025–0.08 mg/kg/dose
  Infants: 0.025–0.1 mg/kg/dose.

Brands: 15 mg Tab; Tilstigmin. 0.5 mg/mL Inj; Myostigmine, Neostigmine.

Nursing Consideration: PO+food. IV doses given in a concentration of 0.5–1 mg/mL and infuse over 2 minutes.

3. Pyridostigmine

Uses: Treatment of myasthenia gravis, reversal of nondepolarizing neuromuscular blocking agents.

Dosage:

- Myasthenia gravis:
  Adults (PO): Initially 60 mg 3 times/day and maintenance range is 60 mg–1.5 g/day. (IM, IV): 2 mg every 2–3 hours
  Children (PO): 7 mg/kg/day in 5–6 divided doses. (IM, IV): 0.05–0.15 mg/kg/dose (Max dose: 10 mg)
- Reversal of nondepolarizing neuromuscular blockade:
  Adults (IV): 10–20 mg.

Brands: 30 and 60 mg Tab; Myestin.

Nursing Consideration: PO+food. IV doses given in a concentration of 0.5 mg/mL over 1 minute for myasthenia and 5 mg/mL over 1 minute for neuromuscular blocking agents.

Chapter

32 Diuretics

Include: (A) Loop diuretics (B) Potassium sparing diuretics
(C) Thiazide and thiazide-like diuretics
(D) Carbonic anhydrase inhibitors (E) Osmotic diuretics

(A) DIURETICS—LOOP DIURETICS

Include: 1. Bumetanide 2. Furosemide 3. Torsemide

Action: Inhibits sodium and chloride reabsorption from the loop of Henle and distal renal tubule thus causing excretion of water and sodium.

Uses: Edema secondary to CHF, hepatic or renal disease, hypertension.

Side Effects: Common side effects are; diarrhea, nausea, tinnitus, dehydration, hypokalemia, hypochloremia, hyponatremia, metabolic alkalosis, hypovolemia. Serious side effects include; renal failure, hearing loss, circulatory collapse.

General Nursing Considerations

- **Assess:** BP and pulse, serum potassium, sodium and chlorine, uric acid, blood glucose, RFT, LFT, daily weight, input and output, fluid status (distribution of edema, skin turgor, lung sounds), signs of electrolyte imbalance (muscle weakness, tingling, numbness, paresthesia, excessive thirst, confusion). Assess for hearing and tinnitus. Determine presence of SLE, drug may worsen condition. When using high doses monitor for hyperlipidemia and hyperuricemia
- **Administration:** PO + food. Give evening dose before 5 pm to prevent disturbance in sleep pattern. Prefer IV over IM. Potentiates the effects of antihypertensives agents, monitor BP
- **Advise:** Take exactly as directed and must be continued even if feeling symptomatically better. Change position slowly to avoid orthostatic hypotension. Always combine additional therapies for hypertension (regular exercises, weight loss, stress control, decrease sodium intake, stop smoking and alcohol). Inform any rapid gain in weight. Diabetic patient should monitor blood glucose levels
- **Desired Outcome:** Control in BP, increased urine output, decreased edema and intracranial pressure as applicable to particular drug.

1. Bumetanide

Dosage:

- Adults (PO): 0.5–2 mg/day divided every 12 hours
  (IM, IV): 0.5–1 mg/dose as needed
- Children and infants (PO, IM, IV): 0.015–0.1 mg/kg/dose every 6–24 hours.

Brands: 1 mg Tab, Bumet.

Nursing Consideration: IV doses can be given undiluted over 1–2 minutes or diluted in D_5W at the rate of 0.25 mg/min.

2. Furosemide

Dosage:

- Adults (PO): 20–80 mg/day once daily
  (IM, IV): 20–40 mg/dose as needed
- Children > 1 month (PO): 1–5 mg/kg/day divided every 6–12 hours
  (IM, IV): 1–2 mg/kg/dose every 6–12 hours
- Hypertension: Adults (PO): 40 mg/dose twice daily.

Brands: 40 mg Tab; Lasix, Tebemid. 10 mg/mL Inj; lasix, FRU.

Nursing Consideration: IV doses can be given undiluted at the rate of 20 mg/min or diluted in 50 mL of D_5W/NS and give at the rate of 4 mg/min.

3. Torsemide

Dosage:

- CHF: Adults (PO, IV): 10–20 mg once daily
- CRF: Adults (PO, IV): 20 mg once daily
- Hepatic cirrhosis: Adults (PO, IV): 5–10 mg once daily
- HT: Adults (PO): 2.5–5 mg once daily.

Brands: 5, 10 and 20 mg Tab; 10 mg/mL Inj. Dytor, Tide.

Nursing Consideration: IV doses can be given undiluted slowly over 3–5 minutes.

(B) DIURETICS—POTASSIUM SPARING DIURETICS

Include: 1. Amiloride 2. Spironolactone 3. Triamterene

Action: Inhibits sodium reabsorption and saving potassium and hydrogen ions in the distal tubule.

Uses: Edema associated with CHF, hepatic cirrhosis; hypertension; primary hyperaldosteronism (spironolactone only).

General Nursing Considerations

- **Assess:** BP, pulse; CBC, serum electrolyte, RFT, LFT, input and output, daily weight, ECG, edema, signs and symptoms of hypokalemia (fatigue, polyuria, polydipsia, weakness, U wave in ECG, arrhythmias), and hyperkalemia (fatigue, muscle weakness, confusion, dyspnea, ECG changes)

- **Administration:** PO + food and give in the morning to prevent nocturnal urination
- **Advise:** Take exactly as advised even if feeling well. Avoid diet rich in vitamin K and sodium. Combine additional therapies for hypertension (HT). Monitor weight and report in case of any major weight gain. They may cause drowsiness, so avoid activities requiring mental alertness.
- **Desired Outcome:** Increase in urine output, decrease in edema and BP, prevent hypokalemia, treatment of hyperaldosteronism as applicable to particular drug.

1. Amiloride

Dosage: PO

- Adults and Children > 20 kg: 5–10 mg/day (Max: 20 mg/day)
- Children 6–20 kg: 0.625 mg/kg/day once daily (Max: 10 mg/day)

Brands: Amiloride + Hydrochlorthiazide: 5+50 mg Tab; Biduret.

Side Effects: Dizziness, arrhythmias, nausea, vomiting, hyperkalemia, hyponatremia, thrombocytopenia.

2. Spironolactone

Dosage: PO

- Adults: Edema, hypokalemia: 25–200 mg/day in divided doses
  HT: 50–100 mg/day in divided doses
  CHF: 25 mg/day
  Diagnosis of primary hyperaldosteronism: 100–400 mg/day in divided doses
- Children: HT, diuretic: 1–2 mg/day in divided doses
  Diagnosis of primary hyperaldosteronism: 100–400 mg/m^2/day in divided doses.

Brands: 25, 100 mg Tab; Aldactone.

Side Effects: Headache, dizziness, erectile dysfunction, gynecomastia. Serious side effects include; agranulocytosis, hyperkalemia.

3. Triamterene

Dosage: PO

- Adults: HT: 100 mg/day divided every 12 hours
- Children: HT: 2–4 mg/kg/day divided every 12 hours.

Brands: 10 mg Tab; Ditide.

Side Effects: Diarrhea, nausea, vomiting, photosensitivity, nephrolithiasis, hemolytic anemia.

Nursing Consideration: Abrupt discontinuation may leads to rebound kaleuresis, so taper off gradually. May cause megaloblastic anemia, supplement FA.

(C) DIURETICS—THIAZIDE AND THIAZIDE-LIKE DIURETICS

Include: 1. Chlorthalidone 2. Hydrochlorothiazide 3. Indapamide 4. Metolazone

Action: Inhibits sodium reabsorption in the distal tubule and increases sodium and water excretion.

Uses: Edema associated with CHF, renal or hepatic diseases; mild to moderate hypertension.

Side Effects: Common side effects are; urinary frequency, dizziness, fatigue, nausea, vomiting, hyperglycemia, hyperuremia, hypokalemia. Serious side effects include; uremia, thrombocytopenia.

General Nursing Considerations

- **Assess:** BP, pulse, serum electrolyte, blood glucose, LFT, RFT, uric acid, input and output, daily weight, edema, signs and symptoms of electrolyte imbalance
- **Administration:** PO + food. Give in the morning to avoid disturbance in night time sleep. Patients resistant to one type of thiazide may respond to another. Stop drug 48 hours before surgery
- **Advise:** Take exactly as directed, even if feeling better. Change position slowly to avoid orthostatic hypotension. Monitor weight daily. Immediately report signs and symptoms of electrolyte imbalance. Comply with additional methods of hypertension control. Avoid alcohol and eat a diet high in potassium
- **Desired Outcome:** Decrease in BP and edema, increase in urine output as applicable to particular drug.

1. Chlorthalidone

Dosage: Adults (PO): 12.5–100 mg once daily.

Brands: 100 mg Tab; Hythalton.

2. Hydrochlorothiazide

Dosage: PO

- Adults: 12.5–100 mg/day divided every 12 hours
- Children > 6 months: 1–3 mg/kg/day divided every 12 hours.

Brands: 12.5 and 25 mg Tab; Aquazide, Thiazide.

3. Indapamide

Dosage: PO

Adults: HT: 1.25–5 mg/day in the morning. Edema: 2.5 mg/day in the morning.

Brands: 1.5 and 2.5 Tab; Lorvas, Natrilix.

4. Metolazone

Dosage: PO

Adults: HT: 2.5–5 mg/day. Edema: 5–20 mg/day.

Brands: 2.5 and 5 mg Tab; Diurem, Metoral.

(D) DIURETICS—CARBONIC ANHYDRASE INHIBITOR

Acetazolamide

Action: Inhibits carbonic anhydrase resulting in decreased secretion of aqueous humor, increased excretion of sodium and water, decreased neuronal discharges from neurons.

Uses: Diuretic, adjunct in treatment of refractory seizures, reduces CSF production in hydrocephalus.

Dosage: PO+food.

- Adults: Epilepsy: 4–16 mg/kg/day in divided doses
  Edema: 250–375 mg/day once daily
- Children: Epilepsy: 4–16 mg/kg/day in divided doses
  Edema: 5 mg/kg/day once daily
- Neonates: Hydrocephalus: 5 mg/kg/dose every 6 hours.

Brands: 250 mg Tab; Acetamide, Diamox.

Side Effects: Common side effects are; anorexia, metallic taste, weakness, weight loss, paresthesias. Serious side effects are; anaphylaxis, hemolytic, and aplastic crisis.

Nursing Consideration:

- **Assess:** CBC, serum electrolyte, blood glucose, input and output, signs and symptoms of hypokalemia, neurological status
- **Administration:** Maintain fluid intake of 2–3 L/day unless contraindicated to prevent stone formation and crytalluria. Avoid high sodium foods
- **Desired Outcome:** Increased diuresis and decrease in seizure frequency.

(E) DIURETICS—OSMOTIC DIURETICS

Mannitol

Action: Increases osmotic pressure of glomerular filtrate which inhibits tubular reabsorption of water and electrolytes.

Uses: Raised ICP and IOP, anuria or oliguria due to ARF.

Dosage: IV

- Adults: Test dose: 12.5 g over 3–5 minutes to produce a urine output of at least 30–50 mL/hr over 2–3 hours
  Initial: 0.5–1 g/kg. Maintenance dose: 0.25–0.5 g/kg every 4–6 hours
- Children: Test dose: 200 mg/kg over 3–5 minutes to produce urine output of at least 1 mL/kg/hr (Max: 12.5 g)
  Initial and maintenance dose: Same as above.

Brands: 100, 350 and 500 mL bottles of mannitol 20% are available.

Side Effects: Common side effects are; nausea, vomiting, headache, thrombophlebitis, electrolyte imbalance. Serious side effects include; convulsions, rebound increase in ICP, acidosis.

Nursing Consideration:

- **Assess:** RFT, serum electrolytes, CVP, vitals, urine output, IOP, neurological status, ICP, signs and symptoms of electrolyte imbalance and dehydration
- **Administration:** Do not refrigerate. Prevent extravasation. IV doses are given undiluted and inline filter should be used for concentration > 20%. Do not give with whole blood. Do not add or mix with other medications
- **Desired Outcome:** Decrease in ICP and IOP, urine output of at least 30–50 mL/hr or increase in urine output.

Chapter

33 Electrolyte Supplements/Minerals

These agents are used for prevention and treatment of deficiencies or excesses of electrolytes and maintenance of normal acid/base balance.

Include:
1. Calcium Gluconate
2. Magnesium Sulfate
3. Potassium Chloride
4. Sodium Bicarbonate
5. Sodium Chloride
6. Zinc Sulfate

1. Calcium Gluconate

Action: Required for transmission of nerve impulses and contraction of cardiac, skeletal and smooth muscles.

Uses: Treatment of hypocalcemia, hyperkalemia, cardiac arrest in the presence of hyperkalemia or hypocalcemia or calcium channel blocking agents.

Dosage: IV: Dosage are expressed in mg or mEq of calcium. 10% solution is equivalent to 9 mg elemental calcium/mL or 0.46 mEq calcium/mL.

- Hypocalcemia: Adults: 2–15 g/day as a continuous infusion or given divided in 3–4 doses. Children and infants: 200–500 mg/kg/day as continuous infusion or in 3–4 divided doses
- Cardiac arrest: Adult: 500–800 mg. Children and infants: 60–100 mg/kg/dose.

Brands: 10% solution for Inj; Calcium gluconate.

Side Effects: Hypotension, bradycardia, arrhythmia, hypercalcemia, hypophosphatemia.

Nursing Consideration:

- **Assess:** Serum, calcium, potassium, magnesium, BP, pulse, ECG, signs and symptoms of hypocalcemia
- **Administration:** For IV use dilute to 50 mg/mL in NS/RL/D_5W and infuse slowly under cardiac monitoring
- **Desired Outcome:** Correction and decrease in signs and symptoms of hypocalcemia.

2. Magnesium Sulfate

Action: It is a cofactor in many enzymatic activity and is required for neurotransmission and muscular excitability.

Uses: Treatment of hypomagnesemia, hypertension, seizures associated with severe eclampsia and acute nephritis.

Dosage: IV: 50% solution in equivalent to 500 mg/mL.

- Hypomagnesemia (IM, IV): Adults: 1 g every 6 hourly for 4 doses
- Children > 1 month: 25–50 mg/kg/dose every 4–6 hours for 3–4 doses
- HT/seizures (IM, IV): Adults: 1 g every 6 hours for 4 doses, children: 20–100 mg/kg/dose every 4–6 hours
- Eclampsia: Adults: 4–5 g as continuous infusion, concurrently with 5 g IM in each buttock, then 4–5 g IM every 4 hours.

Brands: 50% solution for Inj; Magnesium sulfate.

Side Effects: Diarrhea, drowsiness, arrhythmia, bradycardia, hypotension, respiratory depression.

Nursing Consideration:

- **Assess:** Serum magnesium, RFT, input and output, BP, pulse, respiration, neurological status, deep tendon reflexes
- **Administration:** For IM use dilute to 200 mg/mL and give deep into gluteal sites. For IV use dilute in NS/D_5W in a concentration of 50–200 mg/mL and infuse at the rate of 150 mg/min
- **Desired Outcome:** Correction of hypomagnesemia, control of seizures.

3. Potassium Chloride

Action: Major cation of intracellular fluid essential for conduction of nerve impulses; contraction of cardiac, skeletal and smooth muscle.

Uses: Treatment or prevention of hypokalemia.

Dosage: (PO, IV): Potassium chloride contains 13.4 mEq potassium/g

- Prevention of hypokalemia during diuretic therapy: Adults: 20–40 mEq/day in divided doses. Children and infants: 1–2 mEq/kg/day in divided doses
- Treatment of hypokalemia: Adults: 40–100 mEq/day in divided doses. Children and infants: 2–5 mEq/day in divided doses.

Brands: 600 mg Tab; K-card. 1.5 g/15 mL Syp; Keylyte, Potasol. 150 mg Inj; POTCL.

Side Effects: Common side effects are; N/V, abdominal pain, diarrhea, confusion, hypotension, hyperkalemia, paresthesias. Serious is arrhythmias.

Nursing Consideration:

- **Assess:** BP, pulse, ECG, serum potassium, bicarbonate, magnesium, calcium, input and output; signs and symptoms of hypokalemia and hyperkalemia
- **Administration:** For oral use liquid should be diluted in 6–8 parts with water and given slowly. For IV use dilute in NS/RL/D_5W to achieve a concentration of 80 mEq/L for peripheral line use and infuse at the rate of 10 mEq/hr in adults and 0.5 mEq/kg/hr in pediatric patients. IV doses should only be used in patient with adequate urine flow
- **Desired Outcome:** Prevention and correction of serum potassium levels.

4. Sodium Bicarbonate

Action: Dissociates to provide bicarbonate ion which neutralizes hydrogen ions and raises blood and urinary pH.

Uses: Treatment of metabolic acidosis, stabilization of acid-base balance in cardiac arrest, treatment of life-threatening hyperkalemia.

Dosage: (IV): 7.5% solution provide 8.92 mEq/10 mL.

- Cardiac arrest: Adults and children: Initially 1 mEq/kg may repeat with 0.5 mEq/kg in 10 minutes then as indicated by acid base status
- Metabolic acidosis: Adults and children: 2–5 mEq/kg over 4–8 hours, then based on acid base status.

Brands: 7.5% ampule for injection; Sodium bicarbonate.

Side Effects: Gastric distension, edema, metabolic alkalosis, hypernatremia, hypokalemia, hypocalcemia, pulmonary edema.

Nursing Consideration:

- **Assess:** Serum sodium, potassium, calcium, HCO_3, ABG, RFT, input and output, daily weight, edema, lung sounds, signs of acidosis and alkalosis
- **Administration:** For IV use in pediatric patients use the 0.5 mEq/mL solution or dilute the 1 mEq/mL one in SWI. It can be given rapid or slowly as required. Patient should be adequately ventilated before giving in cardiac arrest
- **Desired Outcome:** Clinical improvement in acidosis.

5. Sodium Chloride

Action: Maintains water distribution, fluid and electrolyte balance, osmotic pressure control.

Uses: Treatment of hyponatremia, extracellular volume expansion, restores moisture to nasal membrane, to dilute other medications.

Dosage: Exact dosage depends upon: Clinical status, acid base, fluid and electrolyte balance of patient. 1 liter normal saline contains 154 mEq sodium/L.

- For correction of acute serious hyponatremia:
  mEq Sodium = (desired sodium – actual sodium) × 0.6 × weight in kg. For acute correction use 125 mEq/L as the desired sodium level
- Nasal: Adults and children: as needed.

Brands: 0.9% and 3% sodium chloride solution in 100 and 500 mL packs. 0.9% Nasal Spray; 0.65% gel for nasal application; Nasoclear.

Side Effects: Common side effects are; hypernatremia, hypervolemia, hypokalemia, edema. Serious ones include; CHF, pulmonary edema.

Nursing Consideration:

- **Assess:** Serum sodium, potassium, bicarbonate and chlorine levels, input and output, daily weight, edema, lung sounds, signs and symptoms of hyponatremia or hypernatremia
- **Administration:** Hypertonic (>0.9%) solution should only be used for initial treatment of acute serious symptomatic hyponatremia. Hypertonic normal saline should be given via large vein or central line and maximum rate of infusion in 1 mEq/kg/hr. Use with caution in patients with CHF, HT, renal diseases
- **Desired Outcome:** Prevention or correction of dehydration, correction of serum sodium level.

6. Zinc Sulfate

Action: It is a cofactor for many enzymatic reactions. Required for normal growth and tissue repair, wound healing.

Uses: Prevention and treatment of zinc deficiency, adjunct in diarrhea treatment, to enhance wound healing.

Dosage: PO. Zinc sulfate contains 23% elemental zinc.

Deficiency: Children and infants: 0.5–1 mg elemental zinc/kg/day divided every 12 hours. Adults: 25–50 mg elemental zinc/dose up to 3 times/day.

Brands: 50 mg Tab; Zinconia, Zioral. 20 mg/5 mL Syp; Emzinc, Zincris.

Side Effects: Nausea, vomiting, indigestion, excessive dose may cause hypotension, hypothermia, blurred vision.

Nursing Consideration:

- **Assess:** S. zinc and alkaline phosphatase levels; symptoms of zinc deficiency (growth retardation, impaired wound healing, decreased sense of smell and taste)
- **Administration:** Per oral with food. Do not give along with dairy products
- **Desired Outcome:** Improvement in wound healing, growth; earlier improvement in diarrhea.

Chapter

34 Hematinics and Hematopoietics

Include: (A) Hormones (B) Iron supplements
(C) Vitamins

These drugs either increases quantity or quality of RBC production.

(A) HEMATINICS AND HEMATOPOIETICS—HORMONES

Include: 1. Erythropoietin 2. Nandrolone Decoanate

1. Erythropoietin

Action: Stimulates erythropoiesis (RBC production).

Uses: Anemia of various etiology, e.g. CRF, AZT therapy, prematurity, chemotherapy in patient with nonmyeloid malignancies.

Dosage: Use lowest effective doses and should be adjusted based on response.

- Anemia of CRF: Adults (SC, IV): 50–100 units/kg 3 times/week
  Children (SC, IV): 50 units/kg 3 times/week
- Anemia of AZT therapy: Adults (SC, IV): 100 units/kg 3 times/week for 8 weeks; may be increased to maximum of 300 units/kg
- Anemia of chemotherapy: Adults (SC): 150 units/kg 3 times/week; may be increased after 8 weeks to maximum of 300 units/kg.

Brands: 2000, 3000, 4000, 10000 IU/Vial; Ceriton, Erypro.

Side Effects: Hypertension, convulsions, headache, fever, tachycardia.

Nursing Consideration:

- **Assess:** BP, pulse, RR, input and output, serum electrolytes, RFT, erythropoietin level, serum ferritin, iron and transferrin levels, hematocrit, symptoms of anemia, dietary history, nutritional status
- **Administration:** Not recommended for acute correction of anemia. Always supplement it with blood transfusion and iron therapy. Do not shake vial as it may inactivate glycoprotein and drug; immediately refrigerate unused portion. IV should be given diluted in equal volume of normal saline (NS) over 1–3 minutes. SC route is preferred for patient on dialysis. Erythropoietin may increase the requirement of heparin during hemodialysis. Discontinue therapy if Hb > 12 g% or increase >1 g/dL in 2 weeks period, as it may increase risk of cardiovascular accidents and seizures
- **Advise:** Compliance with dietary restriction, medication and dialysis

- **Desired Outcome:** Reduction in need for BT, increase in Hb%, improvement in anemia symptoms.

2. Nandrolone Decoanate

Action: Stimulates erythropoietin production, also has anabolic effects.

Uses: Anemia of chronic renal failure and chemotherapy; as anabolic in postmenopausal osteoporosis; metastatic breast cancer.

Dosage: Adults (IM)
- Anemia of chemotherapy: 50–150 mg weekly
- Anemia of CRF: 50–200 mg weekly
- As anabolic: 25–100 mg once every 3–4 weeks.

Brands: 25, 50, 100 mg Inj; Deca-durabolin, Nandrobol.

Side Effects: Nausea, diarrhea, insomnia, acne, gynecomastia, virilism, hematuria, hepatic dysfunction.

Nursing Consideration:
- **Assess:** BP, input and output, LFT, serum electrolytes, daily weight, mental status
- **Administration:** Titrate dose, use lowest effective. Do not discontinue abruptly
- **Advise:** Compliance with diet, rest and exercise.

(B) HEMATINICS AND HEMATOPOIETICS—IRON SUPPLEMENTS

Action: Iron is a component of Hb and is required for its production.

Uses: Prevention and treatment of iron deficiency anemia.

Dosage: Either used PO or IV and IM in cases not tolerating oral forms or patient on chronic dialysis or concurrently receiving erythropoietin. Various oral and parenteral forms are available, attention must be paid to the elemental iron available in particular salt.

Oral:
- Adults: Iron deficiency: 120–200 mg/day in divided doses
  Prophylaxis: 60–100 mg/day in divided doses
- Infants and children: Severe deficiency: 4–6 mg elemental iron/kg/day divided 8 hourly
  Mild to moderate deficiency: 3 mg of elemental iron/kg/day divided 8 hourly
  Prophylaxis: 1–2 mg of elemental iron/kg/day divided 8 hourly (Max: 15 mg/day)
- Premature neonates: 2–4 mg elemental iron/kg/day divided 12 hourly (Max: 15 mg/day).

Parenteral:
- Iron sucrose: Adults (IV): Start with a test dose of 50 mg followed by 100 mg given every 1–3 times/week during dialysis for a total dose of 1000 mg; titrate further doses

- Ferric gluconate: Adults (IV): Start with a test dose of 25 mg followed by 125 mg during dialysis; titrate dose based on response
- Children > 6 years (IV): 1 mg/kg during dialysis (Max: 125 mg/dose).

Brands: Fe ammonium citrate 160 mg+B_{12} + FA/15 mL Syp and Cap; Dexorange. Fe ascorbate 100 mg + FA Tab and Fe ascorbate 30 mg/5 mL Syp; Aloha-XT. Fe fumerate 200 mg + FA + B_{12} + Zn Cap; Vartone-Z. Sodium ferric gluconate 62.5 mg Inj; Globac. Iron sucrose 100 mg Inj; Encifer.

Side Effects: Oral: Constipation, dark stool, epigastric pain, diarrhea, nausea, staining of teeth. Parenteral: Serious are; seizures and anaphylaxis. Common are; hypotension, skin staining, urticaria.

Nursing Consideration:

- **Assess:** BP, pulse, hematocrit, transferrin, ferritin, iron level, nutritional status, dietary history, bowel functions
- **Administration:** Avoid in patients receiving frequent BT. PO doses should be given 1 hour prior or 2 hours after meal, if GI discomfort occurs give with meal. Liquid preparations may stain teeths so they should be given diluted in fruit juice or water and administered with straw or place dropper at the back of throat. Do not crush tablet or give with milk or milk products. Discontinue oral iron prior to parenteral iron therapy. Patient should remain lying for 1/2 an hour during parenteral dosing to prevent orthostatic hypotension. Test dose is given diluted in 50 mL of NS and given over 1 hour and remaining portion is given in 100 mL of NS at the rate of 12.5 mg/min if no side effect is seen
- **Advise:** Take as advised. Dark or green stool is normal change. Take diet rich in iron. When treating for iron deficiency anemia treat for additional 3 months after Hb% returns to normal to replenish body iron stores
- **Desired Outcome:** Increase in Hb%, improvement is symptoms of anemia.

(C) HEMATINICS AND HEMATOPOIETICS—VITAMINS

Include: 1. Cyanocobalamin/Vitamin B_{12}
2. Folic acid

1. Cyanocobalamin

Actions: Required for RBC production and hematopoiesis.

Uses: Vitamin B_{12} deficiency, pernicious anemia.

Dosage:

- Adults (PO): Vit. B_{12} deficiency: 100–1000 μg/day
  Pernicious anemia: 1000–2000 μg/day
  (IM): Vit. B_{12} deficiency: 30 μg/day for 5–10 days, then 100–200 μg/month
  Pernicious anemia: 100 μg/day for 6–7 days, then 100 μg/month
- Children (PO): Vit. B_{12} deficiency: 100–1000 μg/day
  (IM): Vit. B_{12} deficiency: 0.2 μg/kg for 2 days, then 1000 μg/day for 2–7 days, then 100 μg/week for 1 month
  Pernicious anemia: 30–50 μg/day for 2 weeks then 100 μg/month.

Brands: Cyanocobalamin 400 μg + FA + Pyridoxin Tab; Hemochek. Cyanocobalamin 15 μg+FA Tab; FAB-12. Cyanocobalamin 500 μg + FA + Nicotinamide 2 mL/Inj; Unifol. Cyanocobalamin 1000 μg + B_1 + B_2 + B_6/3 mL Inj; Optineuron.

Side Effects: Common side effects are; diarrhea, itching, thrombocytosis, headache, heart failure. Serious side effect is anaphylaxis.

Nursing Consideration:
- **Assess:** BP, pulse, RR, CBC, serum potassium, signs of vitamin B_{12} deficiency (pallor, red inflamed tongue, neuropathy, psychosis)
- **Administration:** Per oral with food to increase absorption. PO route has erratic absorption so always use parenteral, unless patient refuses or unable to take IM. Usually given with other vitamins as solitary vitamin B_{12} deficiency is rare
- **Advise:** Stick to well-balanced diet, skin and urine redness seen and may last upto 2–5 weeks during therapy and resolves itself
- **Desired Outcome:** Improvement in anemia, resolution of vitamin B_{12} deficiency symptoms.

2. Folic acid

Action: Required for RBC production.

Uses: Prevention and treatment of megaloblastic anemia and macrocytic anemia; during pregnancy to prevent neural tube defects.

Dosage: PO+food.
- Adults and children > 11 years: 1 mg/day initially then 0.5 mg/day maintenance dose
- Children > 1 year: 1 mg/day initially then 0.1–0.4 mg/day maintenace dose
- Infants: 15 μg/kg/dose daily or 50 μg/day.

Brands: 5 mg Tab; Fol-5, Folet, Folvite.

Side Effects: Irritability, fever, malaise, rashes, bronchospasm.

Nursing Consideration:
- **Assess:** CBC, GI function, signs of megaloblastic anemia (dyspnea, weakness, fatigue), nutritional status, diet
- **Administration:** Usually given with other vitamins as solitary dificiency is rare. Avoid large doses as it may mask the hematologic effects of vitamin B_{12} deficiency
- **Advise:** Take well balanced, vitamin rich diet. Urine may turn intense dark yellow in color
- **Desired Outcome:** Increase in weight, resolution of signs of anemia.

Chapter

35 Hormones

Include:

1. Calcitonin
2. Desmopressin
3. Estrogens
4. Glucagon
5. Insulins
6. Medroxyprogesterone
7. Norethindrone/Norethisterone
8. Oxytocin
9. Progesterone

1. Calcitonin

Action: Inhibits osteoclastic bone resorption and promotes renal excretion of calcium.

Uses: Treatment of Paget's disease of bone, adjunctive therapy for hypercalcemia, management of postmenopausal osteoporosis.

Dosage:

- Postmenopausal osteoporosis: Adults (IM, SC): 100 IU/day. (Intranasal): 200 IU/day in alternate nostrils
- Paget's disease: Adults (IM, SC): Initially 100 IU/day, then 50 IU/day every other days
- Hypercalcemia: Adults (IM, SC): Initially 4 IU/kg every 12 hours (Max: 8 IU/kg every 12 hours).

Brands: 100 IU/mL Vial; Calcynar, Zycalcit. 2200 IU Nasal spray; Miacalcic.

Side Effects: Serious side effect is anaphylaxis. IM, SC: Nausea, vomiting, urinary frequency, rash, swelling. Intranasal: headache, rhinitis, epistaxis, arthralgia.

Nursing Consideration:

- **Assess:** Serum electrolytes and calcium, alkaline phosphatase, urine hydroxyproline(Paget's disease); signs of hypocalcemic tetany; regularly inspect nasal mucosa
- **Administration:** Parenteral: SC is preferred route, if dose is >2 mL then use IM. Give in alternate nostril to decrease irritation
- **Advise:** Report signs of hypocalcemia. Transient flushing and warmth may occur following injection and subsides within 1 hour. Nausea following injection decreases with continuous use. Postmenopausal women should maintain adequate vitamin D and calcium intake. Exercise has been found to arrest and reverse bone loss
- **Desired Outcome:** Decrease calcium level and bone pain. Slowed progression of osteoporosis.

2. Desmopressin

Action: Enhances reabsorption of water in the kidneys; smooth muscle constriction causing vasoconstriction.

Uses: Treatment of primary nocturnal enuresis, diabetes insipidus.

Dosage:

- Nocturnal enuresis ≥ 6 years (Intranasal): 10 μg in each nostril at bedtime. (PO): 0.2–0.6 mg once before bedtime
- Diabetes insipidus:
  Adults (PO): 0.05 mg twice daily. (Intranasal): 0.01–0.04 mg/day as a single or divided doses. (IV, SC): 2–4 μg/day in 2 divided doses
  Children (PO): 0.05 mg daily. Children 3 months–12 years (Intranasal): 0.005– 0.03 mg/day single or in divided doses.

Brands: 0.1 mg Tab; 4 μg/mL Inj; 10 μg nasal spray; Minirin.

Side Effects: Nausea, abdominal cramps, headache, dyspnea, tachycardia, hypotension, hyponatremia.

Nursing Consideration:

- **Assess:** BP, pulse, input and output, weight, urine volume and osmolality, serum osmolality, frequency of enuresis, signs and symptoms of dehydration/water intoxication
- **Administration:** Spray must be primed prior to first use. Begin oral doses 12 hours after last intranasal dose. For IV, dilute to maximum concentration of 0.5 μg/mL and infuse over 15–30 minutes. IV dose is 10 times more potent than intranasal
- **Advise:** Avoid overhydration, blow nose before using spray, notify any headache, dyspnea, heartburn, abdominal pain
- **Desired Outcome:** Decrease in frequency of nocturnal enuresis and urine volume.

3. Estrogens

Include: 1. Estradiol 2. Estrogens (conjugated)

Action: Promote growth and development of female sex organs and maintenance of secondary sex characteristics in women.

Uses: Prevention of postmenopausal symptoms and osteoporosis, female hypogonadism, primary ovarian failure, treatment of atrophic vaginitis.

Dosage: Estrogens should be used in the lowest effective doses and for shortest period of time.

- **Estradiol**

Menopausal symptoms, atrophic vaginitis, osteoporosis, female hypogonadism:

Adults (PO): 0.45–2 mg daily or in a cycle. (IM): 1–5 mg monthly as cypionate or 10–20 mg monthly as valerate. (Gel): as recommended. (Transdermal patch): 50 or 100 μg patch applied twice daily. (Vaginal cream): 2–4 g (0.2–0.4 mg estradiol) daily for 1–2 weeks, then decrease to 1–2 g/day for 1–2 weeks, then maintenance dose of 1 g 1–3 times/week for 3 weeks, then off for 1 week. Then repeat cycle once vaginal mucosa has been restored.

- **Estrogens (conjugated)**

Menopausal symptoms/osteoporosis: Adults (PO): 0.3–1.25 mg daily or in a cycle.
Uterine bleeding: Adults (IM, IV): 25 mg, may be repeated in 6–12 hours if necessary.
Atrophic vaginitis: Adults (PO): 0.3–1.25 mg daily. (Vaginal): 1.25–2.5 mg (2–4 g cream) daily for 3 weeks, off for 1 week, then repeat.

Brands:

- Estradiol: 2 mg Tab; Estrafem. 5 mg/mL Inj; Ethinorm-E (Estradiol benzoate). 10 mg/mL Inj; Progynon depot (Estradiol Valerate). 25, 50, 100 μg patch; Estraderm TTS. 3 mg tube containing 17 b estradiol; E2 Gel. 1 mg/g Gel; Sandrena gel
- Estrogens (conjugated): 0.625 mg Tab; Conjugase, Espauz. 0.625, 1.25 mg Tab; 25 mg Inj; 0.625 mg/1 g vaginal cream; Premarin.

Side Effects: Common side effects are; Nausea, vomiting, weight gain, headache, (women) amenorrhea, dysmenorrhea, edema, hypertension, oily skin, breast tenderness, (men) impotence, testicular atrophy. Serious side effects are; thromboembolism, MI.

Nursing Consideration:

- **Assess:** BP, pulse, LFT, triglycerides and cholesterol levels, serum electrolyte, PT, serum calcium, input and output, daily weight, frequency and severity of menopausal symptoms
- **Administration:** PO, give with food to decrease nausea. For IV use reconstitute with 5 mL of sterile diluent provided and give slowly at the maximum rate of 5 mg/min. Since it contains an oily base, for IM use roll syringe to have uniform dispersion and give deep IM. For vaginal use, use applicator and remain recumbent for at least 30 minutes after application. When transfering from PO to transdermal route, start transdermal therapy after 1 week of last dose. For topical use; apply to clean, dry skin of each thigh in the morning and rub until completely absorbed
- **Advise:** Learn correct method of administration and dose schedule. Do not stop abruptly, it can cause withdrawal bleeding. Report signs and symptoms of fluid retention, thromboembolic disorders, hepatic dysfunction, mental depression. Use sunscreen and protective clothing to prevent skin pigmentation. Regular exercise along with drug can arrest and reverse bone loss in osteoporosis. Go for regular follow up (physical, BP, breast, abdomen, pelvic and Pap smear)
- **Desired Outcome:** Resolution of menopausal symptoms, decreased vaginal and vulvar itching, prevention of osteoporosis.

4. Glucagon

Action: Stimulates hepatic production of glucose. Has positive inotropic and chronotropic effects.

Uses: Acute treatment of severe hypoglycemia. Antidote to beta blockers and calcium channel blockers.

Dosage: IM, IV, SC. (1 unit = 1 mg).

- Hypoglycemia: Adults and children ≥ 20 kg: 1 mg, may be repeated in 15 minutes if required. Children < 20 kg: 0.5 mg or 0.02–0.03 mg/kg, may be repeated in 15 minutes if required
- Antidote to beta blockers: Adults (IV): 50–150 µg/kg followed by 1-5 mg/hr infusion as required
- Antidote to calcium channel blockers: 2 mg.

Brands: 1 mg Inj; Glucagon hypokit.

Side Effects: Common side effects are; Nausea, vomiting, hypotension, respiratory distress. Serious one is anaphylaxis.

Nursing Consideration:

- **Assess:** Blood glucose, serum potassium, signs and symptoms of hypoglycemia, neurological and nutritional status
- **Administration:** Supplement carbohydrate IV or PO specially in patients who lack liver glycogen stores (starvation, malnutrition, adrenal insufficiency). For IV use dilute in SWI for doses > 2 mg and infuse at a rate of 1 mg/min
- **Advise:** Diabetic patients should carry oral glucose. Report signs and symptoms of hypoglycemia
- **Desired Outcome:** Increase in blood glucose level to normal with improved level of consciousness.

5. Insulins

Include: 1. Short-acting insulins 2. Intermediate-acting insulins 3. Long-acting insulins

Action: They lower blood glucose level by increasing glucose uptake, decreased hepatic glucose production.

Uses: Control of hyperglycemia in patients with type 1 and type 2 dibetes mellitus. Only short-acting insulin is used for diabetic ketoacidosis.

Dosage: Depends upon blood glucose level, weight, response, etc.

Short-acting:

- Ketoacidosis (IV): Adults: 0.1 unit/kg/hr as a continuous infusion. Children: loading dose 0.1 unit/kg, then maintenance dose of 0.05–0.2 units/kg/hr as continuous infusion (titrate dose)
- Maintenance therapy (SC): Adults and children: 0.5–1 unit/kg/day.

Intermediate-acting:

- Adults and children (SC): 0.5–1 unit/kg/day.

Long-acting:

- Adults and children > 6 years (SC): Type 2 DM patients: 0.1–0.2 units/kg once daily in the morning or 10 units once or twice daily.

Mixtures:

- Adults and children (SC): 0.5–1 unit/kg/day.

Regular insulin is given within 15–30 minutes before meal. Neutral Protamine Hagedorn (NPH) insulin within 30–60 minutes before meal. Glargine once daily at the same time each day.

Side Effects: Common side effects are; erythema, lipodystrophy, pruritus, swelling. Serious ones include; anaphylaxis, hypoglycemia.

Nursing Consideration:

- **Assess:** BP, pulse, ECG, blood sugar, serum electrolytes, CBC, glycosylated Hb; input and output, daily weight, signs and symptoms of hypoglycemia and hyperglycemia
- **Administration:** Do not interchange insulin as it is available in different types and strengths. Use only insulin syringe for administration and unit marking on syringe must match the insulin units/mL. Do not use if solution is cloudy, discolored or viscous. Rotate vial between palms prior to use to ensure uniform solution. Can be stored at room temperature or in refrigerator for 28 days, do not freeze and keep away from direct sunlight and heat. Rotate injection sites for SC use (thigh, abdominal wall, upper arm). Only regular insulin can be given IV; either direct IV undiluted at the rate of upto 50 units over 1 minute or as a continuous infusion via infusion pump at the rate of 0.05–0.2 units/kg/hr. Mixed insulin should never be used in a pump or for IV infusion. When transferring from once daily NPH insulin to glargine (long-acting) the dose usually remains unchanged but when transferring from twice daily NPH to glargine, the initial dose of insulin glargine is usually reduced by 20%
- **Advise:** Medicine controls but do not cure DM and therapy is life long. Learn technique for administration. Discuss not to change brands, rotate sites; compliance with drug, diet, exercise; regular testing of blood glucose and ketones; signs and symptoms of hypo and hyperglycemia. Should carry source of sugar in case of hypoglycemia, notify doctor if nausea, vomiting or fever develops, blood sugar level not controlled, planning pregnancy
- **Desired Outcome:** Control of blood glucose level without hypo and hyperglycemia.

6. Medroxyprogesterone

Action: Produces secretory changes in the endometrium, histological change in vaginal epithelium, relaxation of uterine smooth muscle, withdrawal bleeding in the presence of estrogen.

Uses: Treatment of secondary amenorrhea and abnormal uterine bleeding caused by hormonal imbalance, advanced unresponsive renal or endometrial carcinoma, pregnancy prevention.

Dosage: Adults.

- Amenorrhea (PO): 5–10 mg/day for 5–10 days
- DUB/induction of menses (PO): 5–10 mg/day for 5–10 days. Start on 16th or 21st day of cycle
- Renal or endometrial carcinoma (IM): 400–1000 mg, may be repeated weekly
- Contraception (IM): 150 mg every 3 months, first dose to be given only during first 5 days of the cycle.

Brands: 2.5 and 10 mg Tab; Deviry, Meprate, Modus. 150 mg/30 mL Inj; Depo-progestin.

Side Effects: Common side effects are; drug induced hepatitis, melasma, chloasma, depression, thromboembolism, thrombophlebitis, breakthrough bleeding, edema, weight gain, bone loss. Serious side effects are; anaphylaxis, angioedema, pulmonary embolism.

Nursing Consideration:

- **Assess:** BP, pulse, respiration, LFT, CBC, serum lipids level, input and output, daily weight, menstrual history, pattern and amount of bleeding
- **Administration:** PO with food to decrease nausea. Shake vigorously before preparing IM dose and if time period between injection is > 14 weeks, see if patient is not pregnant. Parenteral use may lead to bone loss and should not be used for > 2 years. Supplement calcium and vitamin D_3, monitor bone mineral density
- **Advise:** Explain dose schedule, teach breast self-examination, maintain good oral hygiene, report effects like visual changes, incoordination, headache, leg or calf pain, chest pain, breathlessness, edema. Avoid exposure to sunlight to prevent skin pigmentation. Go for regular physical examination, BP, weight monitoring, breast, pelvic and abdominal examination
- **Desired Outcome:** Regularized menstrual period, control of the spread of endometrial or renal cancer.

7. Norethindrone/Norethisterone

For action, side effects and nursing consideration refer to medroxyprogesterone (as above).

Uses: Treatment of amenorrhea, DUB, endometriosis, oral contraceptives.

Dosage: Adolescents and adults (PO):

- DUB/Amenorrhea: As acetate, 2.5–10 mg/day for 5–10 days beginning during the later half of the cycle
- Endometriosis: As acetate, 5 mg/day for 14 days, can be gradually increased upto 15 mg/day
- Contraception: Progesterone only 0.35 mg everyday of the year starting on first day of menstruation.

Brands: 5 mg Tab; Norgest, Regestrone, 200 mg Inj; Noristerat.

8. Oxytocin

Action: Stimulates uterine smooth muscle and produce contractions similar to those seen in spontaneous labor.

Uses: Induction of labor at term, incomplete abortion, postpartum control of bleeding after expulsion of placenta.

Dosage: Adults (IV)

- Induction of labor: 0.5–2 milliunits/min; increase by 1–2 milliunits/min every 15–60 minutes until pattern is established, then decrease the dose
- Postpartum hemorrhage: 10 units infused at a rate of 20–40 milliunits/min
- Incomplete abortion: 10 units at a rate of 20–40 milliunits/min.

Brands: 5 IU/mL Inj; Evatocin, Indox.

Side Effects: Maternal: Common side effects are; hypotension, hypochloremia, hyponatremia, water intoxication, abruptio placentae. Serious side effects are; seizures, coma. Fetal: Common side effects are; hypoxia, arrhythmias. Serious side effects are; ICH, asphyxia.

Nursing Consideration:

- **Assess:** Maternal: BP, pulse, uterine contraction; electrolytes, serum chloride and sodium, fetal heart rate, signs and symptoms of water intoxication. Fetal: Maturity, presentation, pelvic space
- **Administration:** Give IV via infusion pump, dilute 10–20 units in NS/RL to achieve a concentration of 10–20 milliunits/mL and infuse at the rate of 0.05–0.1 mL/min. If contraction occurs < 2 minutes apart, lasting > 60–90 seconds or longer, if there is severe fetal bradycardia or tachycardia then stop infusion and turn patient on her left side to prevent fetal anoxia
- **Desired Outcome:** Contractions similar to menstrual cramp and increase in uterine tone.

9. Progesterone

For action, side effects and nursing consideration refer to medroxyprogesterone (see above).

Uses: Treatment of secondary amenorrhea, abnormal uterine bleeding due to hormonal imbalance. Management of infertility. Support of embryo implantation and early pregnancy.

Dosage:

- Adults (PO): Secondary amenorrhea: 400 mg once daily in the evening for 10 days
- Adults (IM): Secondary amenorrhea: 100–150 mg single dose or 5–10 mg daily for 6–8 days given 8–10 days before expected menstrual period. DUB: 5–10 mg daily for 6 days.

Brands: 100 and 200 mg Cap; 50 mg/mL Inj; Algest, Endogest, Gestone.

Chapter

36 Immunosuppressants

These agents inhibit cell mediated immune response by various mechanisms. Use with caution in patients with infections. While using these agents monitor for infection (vital signs, sputum, stool, urine, WBC). Assess for symptoms of organ rejection throughout therapy. Protect transplant patient from the hospital staff and relatives who may carry infection and better to provide isolation, avoid contact with contagious persons. Transplant patient usually require lifelong therapy to prevent rejection.

Include:
1. Azathioprine
2. Cyclosporin
3. Methotrexate
4. Mycophenolic acid
5. Sirolimus
6. Tacrolimus

1. Azathioprine

Action: Inhibits DNA, RNA and protein synthesis leading to inhibition of mitosis.

Uses: Prevention of transplant rejection, treatment of severe rheumatoid arthritis, SLE, nephrotic syndrome.

Dosage: PO+food to decrease GI discomfort.

Adults and children:

- Transplantation: Initially 2–5 mg/kg/dose once daily, maintenance dose of 1–3 mg/kg once daily
- Rheumatoid arthritis: 1 mg/kg/dose once daily for 6–8 weeks, increase by 0.5 mg/kg every 4 weeks until response is seen.

Brands: 50 mg Tab; Azathioprine, Azimune, Azoran.

Side Effects: Common side effects; anorexia, nausea, vomiting, hepatotoxicity, anemia, leukopenia, thrombocytopenia, chills, fever, alopecia. Serious one is serum sickness.

Nursing Consideration:

- **Assess:** BP, pulse, RFT, LFT, CBC, input and output, daily weight, signs of infection
- **Administration:** For IV use reconstitute 100 mg in 10 mL of SWI/NS/D_5W and infuse over 5 minutes
- **Advise:** Take exactly as advised. If using for rheumatoid arthritis concurrent therapy with salicylates, NSAIDs or corticosteroids are necessary

- **Desired Outcome:** Prevention of transplant rejection, decrease in symptoms of rheumatoid arthritis.

2. Cyclosporin

Action: Inhibits cellular and humoral immune responses.

Uses: Prevention of transplant rejection, treatment of rheumatoid arthritis, severe psoriasis, nephrotic syndrome.

Dosage:

- Prevention of transplant rejection: Adults and children (PO): 14–18 mg/kg/dose 4–12 hours prior to transplant, then 5–15 mg/kg/day divided every 12–24 hours, taper weekly to maintenance dose of 3–10 mg/kg/day. (IV): Initially 5–6 mg/kg/dose 4–12 hours prior to transplant, maintenance dose is 2–10 mg/kg/day in divided doses
- Rheumatoid arthritis: Adults and Children: (PO) Initially 2.5 mg/kg/day in 2 divided doses may be increased upto 4 mg/kg/day slowly.

Brands: 25, 50, 100 mg Cap; Graftin, Imusporin. 50 mg/mL Inj; Sandimmum conc.

Side Effects: Common side effects are; nausea, vomiting, hepatotoxicity, tremor, hypertension, hirsutism, nephrotoxicity, gingival hyperplasia. Serious one is seizures.

Nursing Consideration:

- **Assess:** Vitals, BP, RFT, LFT, CBC, electrolytes, uric acid, lipids, input and output, daily weight, signs and symptoms of infection, hypersensitivity, transplant rejection
- **Administration:** PO+meals. For IV dilute 50 mg in 20–100 mL of NS/D_5W and infuse over 2–6 hours. Do not use plastic for oral doses
- **Advise:** Take exactly as advised. Maintain proper oral hygiene
- **Desired Outcome:** Prevention of transplant rejection, decrease in arthritis symptoms.

3. Methotrexate

Action: Interferes with folic acid metabolism leading to inhibition of DNA synthesis and cell reproduction.

Uses: Treatment of trophoblastic neoplasms, leukemias; breast, head and neck cancer; polyarticular Juvenile Rheumatoid Arthritis, psoriasis.

Dosage:

- Adults: Trophoblastic neoplasma (PO, IM): 15–30 mg/day for 5 days, repeat weekly for 3–5 courses. Head and neck cancer (PO, IM): 25–50 mg/m^2 once weekly
- Children: Antineoplastic dosage range (PO, IM): 7.5–30 mg/m^2/wk or every 2 weeks. (IV): 10–33000 mg/m^2 as bolus or slow infusion.

Brands: 2.5, 7.5 mg Tab; 15 mg/mL Inj; Imutrex, Mexate.

Side Effects: Common side effects are; nausea, vomiting, anorexia, hepatotoxicity, stomatitis, anemia, leukopenia, thrombocytopenia, nephropathy, arachnoiditis. Serious side effects are; pulmonary fibrosis, aplastic anemia.

Nursing Consideration:
- **Assess:** Vitals, BP, LFT, RFT, CBC, urine, uric acid, input and output, daily weight, bleeding, bone marrow depression
- **Administration:** Maintain intensive hydration and urine should be alkalinized before therapy. For IV use reconstitute in 25 mL of NS and administer at a rate of 10 mg/min
- **Desired Outcome:** Improvement of hematopoietic values in leukemia, regression in other cancer.

4. Mycophenolic Acid

Action: Causes suppression of T and B lymphocyte proliferation.

Uses: Prevention of rejection in allogenic renal transplantation.

Dosage: PO on empty stomach 1 hour before or 2 hours after meals.
- Adults: 720 mg twice daily
- Children: 5–16 years: 400 mg/m^2 twice daily.

Brands: 250, 500 mg Tab; Boxmune, Mycophen.

Side Effects: Common side effects are; anorexia, constipation, abdominal pain, anxiety, headache, tremors, edema, hypertension, leukocytosis, leukopenia, thrombocytopenia, dyspnea. Serious one is GI bleeding.

Nursing Consideration:
- **Assess:** BP, pulse, CBC, RFT, LFT, Serum electrolytes
- **Advise:** Inform patient that there is increased risk of lymphoma and other malignancies
- **Desired Outcome:** Prevention of rejection of transplanted organs.

5. Sirolimus

Action: Inhibits T lymphocyte activation and antibody production.

Uses: Prevention of organ rejection in allogenic kidney transplantation.

Dosage: PO±food.

Adults and children ≥ 13 years: 6 mg loading dose followed by 2 mg/day maintenance dose.

Brands: 1 mg Tab; Rapacan.

Side Effects: Hepatotoxicity, rash, insomnia, arthralgias, tremors, leukopenia, thrombocytopenia.

Nursing Consideration:
- **Assess:** BP, Vitals, LFT, RFT, CBC
- **Administration:** Should be taken 4 hours after cyclosporin. Store drug in refrigerator
- **Desired Outcome:** Prevention of transplant rejection.

6. Tacrolimus

Action: Inhibits T lymphocyte activation.

Uses: Prevention of organ rejection in allogenic liver, kidney or heart transplantation, treatment of moderate to severe atopic dermatitis.

Dosage:

- Kidney transplantation:
  Adults (PO): 0.2 mg/kg/day divided 12 hourly. (IV): 0.03–0.1 mg/kg/day in divided doses
  Children (PO): 0.15–0.4 mg/kg/day divided 12 hourly. (IV): 0.03–0.15 mg/kg/day in divided doses
- Atopic dermatitis: Topical
  Adults: Apply 0.03% or 0.1% ointment twice daily
  Children ≥ 2–15 years: Apply 0.03% ointment twice daily.

Brands: 0.5, 1, 2 mg Cap; Pangraf, Tacrograf. 0.03% and 0.1% oint; Olimis, Tacroderm.

Side Effects: Abdominal pain, ascites, raised liver enzymes, headache, tremors, cough, hypertension, nephrotoxicity, electrolyte imbalance, paresthesias. Serious side effects are; anaphylaxis, GI bleeding, seizures.

Nursing Consideration:

- **Assess:** BP, RFT, LFT, electrolytes, CBC, acid base status
- **Administration:** PO is preferred over IV. PO is started 8–12 hours after discontinuation of IV. Therapy is started 6 hours post-transplantation. It should not be used concurrently with cyclosporine. For IV use dilute in NS/D_5W in a concentration of 0.004–0.02 mg/mL and infuse over 24 hours
- **Advise:** Inform patient that there is increased risk of lymphoma and skin cancer
- **Desired Outcome:** Prevention of transplant rejection, management of atopic dermatitis.

Chapter

37 Inotropic/Pressor Agents

Include: 1. Digoxin 2. Dobutamine 3. Dopamine 4. Epinephrine 5. Milrinone 6. Norepinephrine

1. Digoxin

Action: Decreases conduction through SA and AV nodes, prolongs AV node refractory period leading to increased cardiac output and decreased heart rate.

Uses: Treatment of CHF, atrial fibrillation and flutter, SVT.

Dosage: Dosage must be individualized. Dosage required for atrial arrhythmias are higher than those for inotropic effect.

Age	Total digitalizing dose	
	PO	IV
Adults	0.75–1.5 mg	0.5–1 mg
>10 years	10–15 μg/kg	8–12 μg/kg
5–10 years	20–35 μg/kg	15–30 μg/kg
2–5 years	30–40 μg/kg	25–35 μg/kg
1 month–2 year	35–60 μg/kg	30–50 μg/kg

Give half of the digitalizing dose initially then 1/4th at 6 hours and remaining 1/4th at 18 hours intervals. Take ECG after each dose.

Age	Daily maintenance dose	
	PO	IV
Adults	0.125–0.5 mg	0.1–0.4 mg
>10 years	2.5–5 μg/kg	2–3 μg/kg
5–10 years	5–10 μg/kg	4–8 μg/kg
2–5 years	7.5–10 μg/kg	6–9 μg/kg
1 month–2 years	10–15 μg/kg	7.5–12 μg/kg

Daily maintenance dose given is once daily in adults and children >10 years of age. In infants and children <10 years of age it is given divided 12 hourly doses.

Brands: 0.25 mg Tab; Digox, Lanoxin. 0.5 mg/2 mL Inj; Digoxin.

Side Effects: Common side effects are; anorexia, nausea, vomiting, feeding intolerance, fatigue, vertigo, blurred vision, yellow or green vision, bradycardia, hyperkalemia and acute toxicity. Serious one is arrhythmias.

Nursing Consideration:

- **Assess:** BP, ECG, pulse, input and output, daily weight, edema, serum potassium, magnesium, calcium, RFT, LFT
- **Administration:** Before giving loading dose determine whether taken digitalis in the preceding 2–3 weeks, if taken then omit loading dose. Give PO+food. Use caliberated caps and dropper for liquid preparation. Withhold drug if HR< 60 in adults and < 70 in children. IV doses can be given undiluted or diluted 1 mL in 4 mL of SWI/D_5W/NS and given over 5–10 minutes
- **Advise:** Take same time each day. Take HR 2–3 times/day and consult doctor if HR is < 60 or > 100. Do not take antacids or antidiarrheals within 2 hours of digoxin. Do regular follow-up
- **Desired Outcome:** Decrease in severity of CHF, increase in CO, decrease in arrhythmias.

2. Dobutamine

Action: Stimulates β1 adrenergic receptors causing increased contractility and minimal increase in HR.

Uses: Short-term management of heart failure.

Dosage: Adults and children (IV): 2.5–15 μg/kg/min, titrate to desired response.

Brands: 250 mg/5 mL Inj; Dobier, Bouran, Kardia.

Side Effects: N/V, HA, HT, tachycardia, angina, arrhythmia, dyspnea, leg cramps.

Nursing Consideration:

- **Assess:** BP, HR, ECG, input and output, palpate peripheral pulses, appearance of extremities, serum potassium, RFT, PT
- **Administration:** Administer in a large vein. Always correct hypovolemia before drug therapy. For IV use dilute 250–1000 mg in 250–1000 mL NS/D_5W to achieve a concentration of 0.25–5 mg/mL and infuse via infusion devise based on body weight
- **Advise:** Report immediately in case of chest pain, dyspnea, numbness and tingling of extremities, signs of worsening of CHF (increased dyspnea, orthopnea)
- **Desired Outcome:** Increase in cardiac output (CO) and urine output.

3. Dopamine

Action: Stimulates both dopaminergic and adrenergic receptors, the degree of stimulation varies with doses used.

Uses: As an adjunct in the treatment of shock or hypotension to increase CO, BP and urine output.

Dosage: IV: Therapeutic effects are dose dependent.

- **Low doses:** 1–5 μg/kg/min; increases renal blood flow and urine output
- **Intermediate doses:** 5–15 μg/kg/min; increases renal blood flow, HR, cardiac contractility, CO and BP
- **High doses:** >15 μg/kg/min; vasoconstriction, increase in BP.

Brands: 20 mg/mL Inj; Dopacard, Dopacef, Dopaplus.

Side Effects: Nausea, vomiting, headache, dilated pupils, dyspnea, arrhythmias, hypotension.

Nursing Consideration:

- **Assess:** BP, HR, ECG, input and output, palpate peripheral pulses, appearance of extremities
- **Administration:** Correct hypovolemia before starting therapy. If hypotension occurs increase rate of administration. For IV use dilute 200–800 mg in 250–500 mL of NS/D_5W/RL to achieve a concentration of 0.8–3.2 mg/mL and infuse based on body weight via infusion pump. When discontinuing decrease rate gradually to avoid sudden fall in BP
- **Advise:** Report immediately in case of chest pain, dyspnea, numbness and tingling of extremities
- **Desired Outcome:** Increase in BP, urine output, peripheral circulation.

4. Epinephrine/Adrenaline

For details refer to antiasthmatics—adrenergics (Chapter 6).

5. Milrinone

Action: Decreases preload and afterload and increases myocardial contractility.

Uses: Short-term treatment of acute decompensated heart failure.

Dosage: Adults and children (IV): Loading dose of 50 μg/kg, followed by continuous infusion of 0.5 μg/kg/min, titrate to desired effect.

Brands: 1 mg ampule; Myolong. 10 mg ampule; Primacor.

Side Effects: Common side effects are; abnormal LFT, headache, angina/chest pain, hypokalemia, thrombocytopenia. Serious one is ventricular arrhythmias.

Nursing Consideration:

- **Assess:** BP, pulse, ECG; Serum potassium, platelet count, RFT, input and output, daily weight, signs and symptoms of CHF.
- **Administration:** Decrease infusion rate if significant hypotension occurs. For IV use loading dose should be given over 10 minutes in adults and 15 minutes in pediatric patients. For continuous infusion dilute 10 mg in 40 mL of NS/D_5W to achieve a concentration of 200 μg/ml and infuse via infusion pump based on body weight.

6. Norepinephrine/Noradrenaline

Action: Increases cardiac contractility and HR, vasoconstriction.

Uses: Treatment of shock unresponsive to volume replacement, severe hypotension, cardiogenic shock.

Dosage: IV

- Adults: Initially 4 μg/min, then titrate to desired response
- Children: Initially 0.05–0.1 μg/kg/min, then titrate to desired response.

Brands: 4 mg/2 mL Inj; NOR-S.

Side Effects: Vomiting, headache, cardiac arrhythmias, chest pain, dyspnea, increased sweating.

Nursing Consideration: Assess BP, HR, input and output, peripheral perfusion. Administer into large vein. Correct hypovolemia prior to starting therapy.

Chapter

38 Laxatives

Include:

Bulk forming agents	:	Ispaghula
Osmotics	:	Lactulose
Salines	:	Milk of magnesia
Stimulants	:	Bisacodyl
		Sennosides
		Sodium picosulfate
		Tegaserod
Stool softeners	:	Docusate
		Liquid paraffin

Action:

Bulk laxatives: Works by absorbing water and expanding to increase moisture content and bulk in stool.

Osmotics: Increases water content and distention and promotes peristalsis. Lactulose in addition also decreases ammonia levels.

Saline: Draws water into the intestinal lumen.

Stimulants: Act by increasing peristalsis by direct effect on the intestine, alters water and electrolyte secretion; producing net intestinal fluid accumulation and laxation.

Stool softeners: Act by reducing surface tension of the liquid of bowel.

Uses: Prevention and treatment of constipation, preparation of bowel for radiological or endoscopic procedure.

Side Effects: Nausea, abdominal cramps, diarrhea, flatulence.

General Nursing Considerations

- **Assess:** Input and output, electrolytes, bowel function, bowel sounds, abdominal distension, stool color. Stool characeristics whether constipation is present or not. Rule out conditions in which laxatives should not be used
- **Administration:** For morning results better to give at bedtime, always give with plenty of water or juice. More rapid results are seen if taken empty stomach. Do not give within 1 hour of antacids, milk and H_2 antagonists.

Stool softeners and bulk laxatives take many days to show good results. They should not be used in fecal impaction

- **Advise:** Use for only short-term, long-term use may leads to dependence, electrolyte imbalance and bowel tone may be lost. Always take with plenty of liquids (2–2.5 L/day) for better results. Cardiac patients should avoid straining during defecation. Additional measures for good laxation; increase bulk, fluid, exercise, mobility. Laxatives should not be used if there is associated abdominal pain, fever, nausea, vomiting. Tablets should not be chewed. Have a regular schedule for defecation
- **Desired Outcome:** Decrease in constipation. Clearing of confusion, apathy and impaired mental status in case lactulose is used for PSE.

1. Bisacodyl

Dosage:

Adults and Children ≥ 12 years: PO: 5–15 mg/day as single dose

Children 3–12 years: PO: 5–10 mg or 0.3 mg/kg/day as a single dose

Adults and Children ≥ 12 years: RC: 10 mg/day as single dose

Children 3–12 years: RC: 5–10 mg/day as single dose.

Brands: 5 mg Tabs; 5, 10 mg suppositories; Dulcolax.

Nursing Consideration: Lubricate suppositories before insertion and can be given 15–30 minutes before bowel movement is desired.

2. Docusate

Dosage:

- Adults and older children: RC: 50–100 mg as required
- Adults and Children ≥ 12 years: PO: 50–400 mg/day in 1–4 divided doses
- Children < 3 years: PO: 10–40 mg/day in 1–4 divided doses
- Children 3–12 years: PO: 20–60 mg/day in 1–4 divided doses.

Brands: 100 mg Tabs; 50 mg/5 mL syp; 0.25% enema; Laxicon.

3. Ispaghula

Dosage: Adults: PO: 3–12 g/day of refined husk in divided doses.

Brands: 3.5 g/5 g; Evaq, Fibrodiet, Igol.

Nursing Consideration: Take with plenty of fluids.

4. Lactulose

Uses: In addition also used for portal systemic encephalopathy (PSE).

Dosage: PO

- Constipation: Adults: 10–20 g/day (15–30 mL) once or divided doses
Children: 5 g/day (7.5 mL) once or divided doses
- PSE: Adults: 20–30 g (30–45 mL) 3–4 times/day.
Children: 2.5–40 mL/day in divided doses.

Brands: 3.33 g/5 mL liquid; Duphalac, Laxil, Looz.

Nursing Consideration: Assess mental status prior and during therapy in PSE. Monitor serum electrolyte level in chronic therapy. Blood sugar levels may be raised in diabetic patients.

5. Liquid Paraffin and Milk of Magnesia

Dosage: PO

- Milk of Magnesia: Adults: 30–60 mL single or divided doses
  Children: 6–12 years: 15–30 mL single or divided doses
  2–5 years: 5–15 mL single or divided doses.
- Liquid Paraffin: As this is available in combination calculate as per milk of magnesia doses.

Brands: Milk of magnesia 3.75 mL + Liquid paraffin 1.25 mL/5 mL susp; Cremaffin, Duolaxin, Trulax.

6. Sennosides

Dosage: PO

- Adults and Children ≥ 12 years: 12–50 mg 1–2 times/day
- Children 6–12 years: 6–25 mg 1–2 times/day
- Children 2–5 years: 3–12.5 mg 1–2 times/day.

Brands: 12 mg Senna extract (as cal. salts) per tablet; Senade, Senasof.

Nursing Consideration: May discolor urine and feces to yellow, pink, red.

7. Sodium Picosulfate

Dosage: Adults: PO: 5–10 mg at bedtime.

Brands: 10 mg tabs; Cremalax, Fecolax. 5 mg/5 mL Syp; Coso, Laxkair.

8. Tegserod

Dosage: Adults: PO: 3–6 mg twice before meals.

Brands: 2, 6 mg Tabs; Tegibis, Ibsinorm.

Chapter

39 Lipid Lowering Agents

Include: (A) HMG-CoA reductase inhibitors:

1. Atorvastatin
2. Lovastatin
3. Pravastatin
4. Rosuvastatin
5. Simvastatin

(B) Miscellaneous:

1. Ezetimibe
2. Fenofibrate
3. Gemfibrozil

General Nursing Considerations

- **Assess:** Serum cholesterol, triglycerides level, LFT, CK, CPK, dietary record, fat and alcohol consumption, weight
- **Administration:** Try dietary therapy for 2–3 month before starting drug therapy. If liver enzymes and CK is elevated, avoid using drugs
- **Advise:** Should be used along with diet restriction, exercises and cessation of alcohol. Report muscle pain, tenderness, weakness, especially with fever or malaise
- **Desired Outcome:** Decrease in cholesterol and triglycerides level, increase in HDL, slowing the progression of coronary artery disease.

(A) HMG-CoA REDUCTASE INHIBITORS

Action: Inhibits HMG-CoA reductase enzyme involved in cholesterol synthesis.

Uses: Hyperlipidemia.

Dosage:

- Atorvastatin: Adults: PO: 10–20 mg once daily in the evening
  Children 10–17 years: PO: 10 mg/day (Max: 20 mg/day)
- Lovastatin: Adults: PO: 20–40 mg once daily with evening meal
- Pravastatin: Adults: PO: 40 mg once daily at bedtime
  Children 8–18 years: PO: 20–40 mg once daily
- Rosuvastatin: Adults: PO: 5–20 mg once daily
- Simvastatin: Adults: PO: 5–80 mg once daily in the evening
  Children 10–18 years: PO: 10 mg once daily.

Brands:
- Atorvastatin: 5, 10, 20, 40 mg Tabs; Atocor, Atorlip
- Lovastatin: 10, 20 mg Tabs; Lotin, Lovex
- Pravastatin: 10, 20 mg Tabs; Prastatin, Pravator
- Rosuvastatin: 5, 10, 20 mg Tabs; Novastat, Rosuvas
- Simvastatin: 5, 10, 20 mg Tabs; Satin, Simvas.

Side Effects: Diarrhea, heartburn, flatus, abdominal cramps, constipation, blurred vision, rashes, hepatitis, rhabdomyolysis.

(B) MISCELLANEOUS

1. Eztimibe

Action: Inhibits absorption of cholesterol in the small intestine.

Uses: Hypercholesterolemia, dyslipidemias.

Dosage: Adults: PO: 10 mg once daily+meals. Avoid with antacids, reduces drug effect.

Brands: 10 mg Tabs; Mibe, Zetica.

Side Effects: Nausea, cholecystitis, cholelithiasis.

2. Fenofibrate

Action: Inhibits triglyceride synthesis.

Uses: Hypercholesterolemia, dyslipidemias.

Dosage: Adults: PO: 50–150 mg once daily ± meals.

Brands: 160 mg Tabs; 200 mg Cap; Fenacor, Lipicard.

Side Effects: Weakness, pancreatitis, cholelithiasis.

3. Gemfibrozil

Action: Decreases production of triglycerides and triglycerides carrier protein, increases HDL.

Uses: Hyperlipidemia.

Dosage: Adults: PO: 600 mg twice daily half an hour before breakfast and dinner.

Brands: 300 mg Cap; Gempar, Lopid.

Side Effects: Diarrhea, epigastric pain, anemia, blurred vision.

Chapter

40 Neuromuscular Blocking Agents

Include: 1. Atracurium 2. Pancuronium 3. Succinylcholine 4. Vecuronium

Action: Acts by inhibiting transmission of nerve impulses by binding with cholinergic receptor sites.

Uses: Eases endotracheal intubation as an adjunct to general anesthesia and relaxes skeletal muscle during surgery or mechanical ventilation.

Side Effects: Common side effects are; bradycardia, decreased motility, excess salivation, rash, erythema. Serious side effects are; apnea, bronchospasm, cyanosis, respiratory depression.

General Nursing Considerations

- **Assess:** Pulse, respiration, ECG, airway, serum electrolytes, CBC, RFT, LFT, input and output, urinary retention, frequency, hesitancy, recovery pattern
- **Administration:** Use nerve stimulator to determine neuromuscular blockage. Anticholinesterase are used to reverse blockage. Use anesthesia/analgesia concurrently with blocking agents. If eyes remains open during procedure protect cornea with artificial tears. Administer in a closely monitored setting and only when intubated
- **Advise:** As consciousness is not impaired by blocking agents explain all procedure to patient without general anesthesia. Reassure that communication will return to normal as medication effect weans off
- **Desired Outcome:** Paralysis of jaw, eyelid, head, neck and rest of body. Better compliance with mechanical ventilation
- **Treatment of overdose:** Use edrophonium or neostigmine; atropine.

1. Atracurium

Dosage: IV

- Adults and children >2 years: Initially 0.4–0.5 mg/kg then 0.08–0.1 mg/kg 30–45 minutes later to maintain block
- Neonates, infants and children ≤2 years: Initially 0.3–0.4 mg/kg followed by maintenance dose of 0.3–0.4 mg/kg as needed

Brands: 10 mg/mL Inj; Artacil, Tracrium

Nursing Consideration: IV doses can be given undiluted over 5 minutes or diluted in NS/D_5W in a concentration of 0.5 mg/mL as continuous infusion.

2. Pancuronium

Dosage: IV

- Adults: 0.15 mg/kg every 30–60 minutes as needed
- Infants and children: 0.1 mg/kg every 30–60 minutes as needed.

Brands: 2 mg/mL Inj; Fancuron, Pavulon.

Nursing Consideration: IV doses can be given undiluted or diluted in D_5W/NS/RL in a concentration of 0.01–0.08 mg/mL as continuous infusion. Store in a refrigerator and do not store in plastic syringes.

3. Succinylcholine

Dosage:

- Adults (IV, IM): Pretreatment with atropine may reduce chances of bradycardia. Initially 0.6 mg/kg, maintenance dose is 0.04–0.07 mg/kg every 5–10 minutes as needed
- Children (IV): Initially 1–2 mg/kg, maintenance dose is 0.3–0.6 mg/kg every 5–10 minutes as needed. (IM): 2.5–4 mg/kg.

Brands: 50 mg/mL Inj; Scolax, Scoline.

Nursing Consideration: IV doses can be given undiluted or diluted in NS/D_5W in a concentration of 1–2 mg/mL.

4. Vecuronium

Dosage: IV

- Adults and children > 1 year: 0.1 mg/kg/dose, may be repeated every hour as needed.

Brands: 2 mg/mL Inj; Neovec, Vecuron.

Nursing Consideration: IV doses can be given diluted in NS/RL/D_5W in a concentration of 1–2 mg/mL.

Chapter

41 Sedatives/Hypnotics

Action: These agents cause generalized CNS depression.

Uses: Used to provide sedation before procedures and to manage insomnia. Some agents are used for multiple indications.

General Nursing Considerations

- **Assess:** BP, pulse, respiratory status, mental status, insomnia and seizure pattern. Assess drowsiness, ataxia or visual disturbances, they may require dose adjustment
- **Administration:** Should not be used in comatose, uncontrolled severe pain and those with pre-existing CNS depression. Create environment for sleep (quite dark room, no disturbances, soothing colors, decrease day time sleep). Withdraw slowly to prevent withdrawal symptoms. Give most of the daily dose at bedtime, with smaller doses during waking hours
- **Advise:** Chronic therapy may cause physical and psychological dependence. Avoid alcohol, tobacco, other CNS depressants. Advise psychotherapy. Report any suicidal tendencies, signs of increased depression immediately
- **Desired Outcome:** Good sleep, sedation, seizure control as applicable to particular drug.

(A) SEDATIVES/HYPNOTICS—BARBITURATES

Include: Phenobarbital.

For details refer to anticonvulsants section (Chapter 10) and main discussion.

(B) SEDATIVES/HYPNOTICS—BENZODIAZEPINES

Include:

1. Chlordiazepoxide
2. Diazepam
3. Flurazepam
4. Lorazepam
5. Midazolam
6. Oxazepam
7. Temazepam
8. Triazolam

1. Temazepam

Uses: Insomnia, anxiety.

Dosage: Adults (PO): 7.5–30 mg at bedtime.

Brands: 7.5, 15, 30 mg Cap; Restoril.

Side Effects: Hangover, constipation, blurred vision, dizziness.

2. Triazolam

Uses: Insomnia.

Dosage: Adults (PO): 0.125–0.25 mg at bedtime.

Brands: 0.125, 0.25 mg Tab; Halcion.

Side Effects: Dizziness, hangover, headache, sedation, blurred vision.
* For details of other drugs refer to anticonvulsants section (Chapter 10).

(C) SEDATIVES/HYPNOTICS—MISCELLANEOUS

Far actions and nursing consideration refer main discussion.

1. Chloral Hydrate

Uses: Short-term nocturnal and preoperative sedation.

Dosage:
- Adults (PO): 250 mg 3 times/day. (RC): 20–50 mg
- Children > 1 month (PO/RC): 20–50 mg/kg/day divided every 8 hours.

Brands:

Side Effects: Excess sedation, diarrhea, tolerance, nausea, vomiting.

2. Zaleplon

Uses: Insomnia.

Dosage: Adults (PO): 5–20 mg at bedtime.

Brands: 5,10 mg Cap; Zalpilo, Zaplon.

Chapter

42 Skeletal Muscle Relaxants

Include: Centrally acting: Baclofen
Carisoprodol
Chlorzoxazone
Methacarbamol
Tizanidine
Direct acting: Dantrolene

Action: Centrally acting agents acts at spinal level by inhibiting reflexes. Direct acting agents act on skeletal muscles.

Uses: Baclofen and Tizanidine are used for treatment of spasticity associated with CP, reversible spasticity associated with multiple sclerosis or spinal cord lesions. Other agents are used for muscle spasm and pain associated with musculoskeletal conditions. Dantrolene is used for spasticity associated with spinal cord lesions, stroke, cerebral palsy, multiple sclerosis

Side Effects: Common side effects are; dizziness, fatigue, weakness, nausea, anorexia, hypotension. Serious side effects include; GI bleeding, anaphylaxis.

General Nursing Considerations

- **Assess:** Input and output, LFT, RFT, pain, stiffness, range of movement before and during therapy. Extent of musculoskeletal/neurological disorders associated with muscle spasm; any seizure or history of seizure (may cause loss of seizures control)
- **Administration:** Monitor BP, HR during parenteral administration. Give with milk or food to decrease GI irritation. Do not stop abruptly. They may cause psychological dependence. Determine lowest dose effective to treat
- **Advise:** Use additional therapies (rest, yoga, physical therapy, heat). Avoid activities requiring alertness. Change position slowly to prevent orthostatic hypotension. Avoid alcohol and other CNS depressants. Increase bulk and fluids to prevent constipation
- **Desired Outcome:** Decrease in muscle spasm and pain, and increase in range of movement.

1. Baclofen

Dosage:

- Adults and Children ≥ 12 years: PO: 5 mg 3 times/day, may be increased every 3 days to maximum of 80 mg/day. IT: 300-800 μg/day
- Children < 12 years: PO: 10–15 mg/day divided every 8 hours, may be increased every 3 days to maximum of 40 mg/day. IT: 100–300 μg/day.

Brands: 10, 25 mg Tabs; 50 μg/mL Inj; Liofen.

Nursing Consideration: For intrathecal use, test dose should be used first. This drug is known to decrease seizure threshold.

2. Carisoprodol

Dosage: Adults: PO: 250–350 mg 4 times/day for not more than 2–3 weeks.

Brands: 350 mg Tabs; Carisoma.

Nursing Consideration: Idiosyncratic reactions, anaphylaxis may occur within minutes to hour of first dose.

3. Chlorzoxazone

Dosage: PO

- Adults: 250–750 mg 3–4 times/day
- Children: 20 mg/kg/day divided every 6–8 hours.

Brands: Available in combination. Chlorzoxazone 500 mg + Diclofenac 50 mg + paracetamol 500 mg: Tabs; Megadol SP, Mobizox.

4. Dantrolene

Dosage: PO

- Adults: 25 mg/day initially, may be increased every 4–7 days to maximum of 400 mg/day in divided doses
- Children: Initial, 0.5 mg/kg/dose divided 12 hourly and can be increased every 4–7 days to maximum of 3 mg/kg/dose.

Brands: 25, 50, 100 mg cap; Dantrium.

5. Methacarbamol

Dosage:

- Adults: PO: 1.5 g 4 times/day. IM, IV: 1–3 g/day for maximum of 3 days
- Children: IV: For tetanus: 15 mg/kg dose for 3 days only.

Brands: 500 mg Tabs; 100 mg/mL Inj; Robinax.

6. Tizanidine

Dosage: PO

Adults: 4 mg every 6–8 hours initially, can be increased gradually to a maximum of 24 mg/day.

Brands: 2, 4 mg Tabs; Tizan.

Chapter

43 Thrombolytics

Include: 1. Alteplase
2. Streptokinase
3. Urokinase

Action: Acts by converting plasminogen to plasmin, which then degrades fibrin, fibrinogen, etc. in the clot into soluble fragments.

Uses:

- Alteplase: Acute ischemic stroke, MI, pulmonary embolism
- Streptokinase: Pulmonary embolism, MI, deep vein thrombosis, occluded cannulae, arterial thromboembolism
- Urokinase: Acute massive pulmonary embolism.

Side Effects: Common side effects are; decreased hematocrit, urticaria, headache, nausea, hypotension, dyspnea. Serious side effects are; gastro intestinal, genitourinary, intracranial and retroperitoneal bleeding, anaphylaxis.

General Nursing Considerations

- **Assess:** HR, BP, RR and status, peripheral pulse, ECG, bleeding, neurological status, temperature, extremities for perfusion before and during therapy. Lab tests; Hb%, platelet, FDP, PT, APTT, BT, CV status, history of hypertension or chest pain/or stroke symptoms
- **Administration:** Not effective for thrombi over 1 week old, so begin therapy as soon as possible. Keep emergency drugs ready during therapy. Avoid IM injections and arterial punctures. Give heparin following therapy to prevent reocclusion. Premedicate with antiemetic to prevent nausea, vomiting. To prevent bruising avoid unnecessary handling of client. Use FFP or cryoprecipitate for bleeding
- **Advise:** Strict bedrest, avoid injury (injury prone activities, shaving, vigorous tooth-brushing) during therapy
- **Desired Outcome:** Restoration of blood flow and catheter patency, prevention of neurological sequel in acute ischemic stroke.

1. Alteplase

Dosage:

- Adults: IV
  Acute MI: Accelerated infusion: 15 mg bolus, then 0.75 mg/kg over 30 minutes, then 0.5 mg/kg over next 60 minutes 3 hours infusion: 1.25 mg/kg given over 3 hours (total: 100 mg)
  Acute ischemic stroke: 0.9 mg/kg given as infusion over 1 hour
  Pulmonary embolism: 100 mg over 2 hours
- Adults and Children > 30 kg: IV: 2 mg/2 mL instilled into occluded catheter
- Adults and Children < 30 kg: IV: 1 mg/1 mL instilled into occluded catheter.

Brands: 50 mg/vial, Actilyse.

Nursing Consideration: For IV dissolve in solvent water in a concentration of 0.5–1 mg/mL.

2. Streptokinase

Dosage: Adults: IV

- MI: 1.5 million units given as a continuous infusion over 60 minutes
- Deep vein thrombosis, pulmonary and arterial embolism: 250,000 units loading dose over 30 minutes followed by 100,000 units/hr for 24 hours for pulmonary or arterial embolism and 72 hours for deep vein thrombosis.

Brands: 7.5 and 15 lac IU/vial; Eskinase, Prokinase, Streptase.

Nursing Consideration: For IV dilute in NS/D_5W, maximum concentration is 1.5 million units/50 mL.

3. Urokinase

Dosage: Adults: IV: 4400 units/kg loading dose followed by 4400 units/kg/hr for 12 hours.

Brands: 2.5, 5.0, 7.5 lac IU/vial; Dukinase, Uropase.

Chapter

44 Thyroid Hormones

Include: 1. Levothyroxine 2. Liothyronine

Action: Replacement in hypothyroidism to restore normal hormonal balance.

Uses: Hypothyroidism.

Side Effects: Seen with overdoses. Cramps, diarrhea, dyspnea, nervousness, headache, chest pain, arrhythmias, increased sweating, hair and weight loss.

Nursing Consideration:

- **Assess:** Thyroid function test, blood and urine glucose, pulse, BP, ECG, height and weight, psychomotor development in children, signs and symptoms of hypothyroidism and hyperthyroidism
- **Administration:** Give as single dose before breakfast. Initiate treatment with small doses that are gradually increased. A child dosage may be the same as the dosage for an adult
- **Advise:** Take exactly as directed. Medication only controls hypothyroidism and therapy is lifelong. Do not change brand. Avoid iodized salt, saltwater fish/ shellfish, cabbage, multivitamin with high iodine content. Monitor growth in children
- **Desired Outcome:** Resolution of signs and symptoms of hypothyroidism.

1. Levothyroxine

Dosage: PO

- Adults: Initially 50 μg once daily, then can be increased slowly to maintenance dose of 75–125 μg/day
- Children ≥ 12 years: 2–3 μg/kg/dose. 6–12 years: 4–5 μg/kg/dose. 1–5 years: 5–6 μg/kg/dose. 6–12 months: 6–8 μg/kg/dose. 3–6 months: 8–10 μg/kg/ dose.

Brands: 25, 50, 100, 125 μg Tab; Thyronorm, Thyrochek.

2. Liothyronine

Dosage:

- Adults (PO): Mild hypothyroidism: 25 μg once daily. Myxedema: 2.5–5 μg once daily may be increased upto 25 μg/day slowly
- Adults (IV): Myxedema coma: Initially 25–50 μg/day
- Children (PO): Initially 5 μg/day, may be increased by 5 μg every 3 days to maximum of 20 μg/day for < 1 year; 50 μg/day for 1–3 years and 75 μg/day for > 3 years

Brands: 20 μg Tab; Tetroxin. 20 μg Inj; Triiodothyronine.

Chapter 45

Vaccines

Include:

1. BCG
2. DPT
3. DT
4. Hemophilus influenzae
5. Hepatitis-A
6. Hepatitis-B
7. Human papillomavirus
8. Influenza virus
9. IPV
10. Measles
11. MMR
12. Meningococcal
13. OPV
14. Pneumococcal
15. Rabies
16. Rotavirus
17. Td
18. TT
19. Typhoid
20. Varicella

1. BCG (Bacille Calmette-Guérin)

Uses: Prevention of primary tuberculosis.

Dosage: Give 0.1 mL ID, single dose from birth to 6 weeks.

Brands: 10 dose BCG Vial by Aventis and Serum.

Nursing Consideration: Vial is to be reconstituted in 1 mL of diluent provided with vaccine and use within 4 hours of reconstitution. Preferred site: left deltoid region.

2. DPT (Diphtheria, Pertussis, Tetanus)

Uses: Active immunization against DPT upto 5 years of age.

Dosage: 0.5 mL deep IM, anterolateral region of upper thigh. Primary doses given at 6, 10, 14 weeks and booster doses at 18 months and 5 years.

Brands: Whole cell single and multidose Vial; Triple antigen. Acellular 0.5 mL single dose Inj; Infanrix, Tripacel.

Nursing Consideration: Shake well before withdrawal into syringe. Do not use if precipitate is present. Acellular vaccine has lower incidence of side effects.

3. DT (Diphtheria, Tetanus)

Uses: Active immunization of children where pertussis component is contraindicated.

Dosage: 0.5 mL deep IM, anterolateral region of upper thigh.

Brands: Single and multidose Vial; Dual antigen.

Nursing Consideration: Shake well before use, do not use if precipitate is seen.

4. *Hemophilus influenzae* Type-B Conjugate

Uses: Active immunization against Hemophilus type-B.

Dosage: 0.5 mL deep IM, anterolateral aspect of upper thigh. Three primary doses when started below 6 months, 2 doses between 6–12 months and 1 dose between 12–18 months. Single booster dose is given between 15–18 months. When started after 18 months to 5 years then single primary dose is given. Keep a gap of 4 weeks between doses.

Brands: 0.5 mL single dose Vials; Hiberix, Act-hib, Hibpro.

Nursing Consideration: Always use diluent provided with the pack.

5. Hapatitis-A

Uses: Active immunization of children and adults against hepatitis-A.

Dosage: IM, deltoid area. Given after 1 year of age in two primary doses at 6 months intervals.

Brands: 720 (Ped) ELISA units/0.5 mL and 1440 (adults) ELISA units/1 mL; Havrix. 80 U (Ped)/0.5 mL and 160 (adults)/1 mL Inj; Avaxim.

6. Hepatitis-B

Uses: Active immunization of adults and children against hepatitis-B.

Dosage: IM. Anterolateral aspect of upper thigh in children and deltoid in adults.

- Children: 10 µg or 0.5 mL. Primary doses at birth, 6, 14, weeks or 6, 10, 14 weeks or 0, 1, 6 months
- Adults: 20 µg or 1 mL. Primary doses at 0, 1, 6 months or 0, 1, 2 months

Brands: Single and multidose Vial; Bevac, Engerix-B, Genevac-B.

Nursing Consideration: Shake well before use, do not use if precipitate is seen.

7. Human Papillomavirus Vaccine

Uses: Prevents cervical carcinoma precancerous genital lesions and genital warts.

Dosage: IM. Recommended after 9 years of age. Deltoid or upper thigh. Three doses at 0, 2, 6 months.

Brands: 0.5 mL single dose Vial; Gardasil.

8. Influenza Virus Vaccine

Uses: Active immunization during epidemic or routinely in children.

Dosage: IM. Anterolateral aspect of upper thigh in < 3 years and in deltoid > 3 years of age.

- 6 month–35 months: 0.25 mL, 2 doses at 4 weeks interval followed by single dose annually

- 3–8 years: 0.5 mL, 2 doses at 4 weeks interval followed by single dose annually.
  ≥ 9 years and adults: 0.5 mL single dose annually.

Brands: 7.5 µg of A + 7.54 µg of B Virus antigen/0.25 mL Inj; Vaxigrip.

9. IPV (Inactivated Polio Vaccine)

Uses: Active immunization against type 1, 2, 3 polio in all children upto 5 years of age.

Dosage: IM, 0.5 mL. 3 primary doses at 6, 10, 14 weeks or 8, 12, 16 weeks; booster at 15 months.

Brands: 0.5 mL Inj; Imovax, Polprotec.

10. Measles

Uses: Active immunization of all children of 7–9 months age group.

Dosage: SC, 0.5 mL over upper arm.

Brands: 0.5 mL Inj; M-Vac.

11. MMR

Uses: Active immunization of all children against measles, mumps and rubella after 15 months of age.

Dosage: SC, 0.5 mL over upper arm.

Brands: 0.5 mL Inj; Tresivac, Priorix.

12. Meningococcal Vaccine

Uses: Active immunization against *N. meningitidis* infection during epidemic.

Dosage: IM, 0.5 mL. Given in children > 2 years of age during epidemic single dose followed by booster every 2 years.

Brands: 0.5 mL Inj; Mancevax, Meningococcal.

13. OPV (Oral Polio Vaccine)

Uses: Active immunization against type 1, 2, 3 polio in all children under 5 years of age.

Dosage: PO, 2 drops at brith, 6, 10, 14 weeks; booster at 18 months and 5 years.

Brands: 20 doses OPV Vial by Haffkine and GSK.

14. Pneumococcal Vaccine

Uses: Active immunization against pneumococcal infection.

Dosage: IM/SC, 0.5 mL.

- 23 Valent is recommended in > 2 years of age, single primary dose followed by booster after 3–5 years
- For 7 valent, 3 primary doses are given at 6, 10, 14 weeks followed by booster at 12–15 months.

Brands: 0.5 mL Inj; Pneumo-23 (23 valent), Prevenar (7 valent).

15. Rabies Vaccine

Uses: Pre-exposure prophylaxis in high-risk group and postexposure prophylaxis after exposure to rabied animals.

Dosage: IM, 0.5 mL.

- Pre-exposure prophylaxis: Three doses at 0, 7 and 28 days
- Postexposure: Six doses at 0, 3, 7, 14, 28 and 90 days.

Brands: 0.5 mL Inj; Rabipur, Rabivax, Verorab.

16. Rotavirus Vaccine

Uses: Active immunization to prevent rotavirus gastroenteritis.

Dosage: PO, 2 doses at 4 weeks interval starting at 6 weeks of age.

Brands: 1 mL dose; Rotarix.

17. Td

It is a low dose diphtheria vaccine combined with tetanus toxoid.

Dosage: IM, 0.5 mL. Recommended in > 7 years of age and should replace TT at 10 and 16 years age.

Brands: 0.5 mL Inj; Td vac.

18. TT (Tetanus Toxoid)

Uses: Active immunization against tetanus in children and adults, antenatal immunization after 5 months of pregnancy.

Dosage: IM, 0.5 mL. Two doses at 8 weeks interval during pregnancy and single dose in other conditions.

Brands: 0.5 mL ampule; BETT.

19. Typhoid Vaccine

Uses: Active immunization of all and in endemic area.

Dosage: IM, 0.5 mL after 2 years of age. Single primary dose followed by booster every 3 years.

Brands: 0.5 mL Inj; Biovac, Typbar, Typhim-Vi.

20. Varicella/Chickenpox Vaccine

Uses: Active immunization against varicella in healthy subjects and susceptible healthy close contacts.

Dosage: 0.5 mL, SC. Single dose in 1–13 years of age group and 2 doses 4 weeks apart in >13 years of age.

Brands: 0.5 mL Inj; Varivax, Okavax.

Chapter

46 Vitamins

Include: (A) Fat-soluble vitamins
(B) Water-soluble vitamins

General Nursing Considerations

- **Assess:** Nutritional status, dietary history by recall, signs and symptoms of particular vitamin deficiency
- **Administration:** Multivitamin combination is preferred as solitary vitamin deficiency is usually rare. Prefer oral preparations over parenteral unless indicated or patient not willing or unable to take orally. Do not use mineral oil while using fat-soluble vitamins
- **Advise:** Take well-balanced and vitamin rich diet
- **Desired Outcome:** Decrease in the signs and symptoms of vitamin deficiency and improvement in well-being.

(A) FAT-SOLUBLE VITAMINS

Include: 1. Vitamin-A
2. Vitamin-D
3. Vitamin-E
4. Vitamin-K

For general nursing considerations of each drug refer to main discussion (see above).

1. Vitamin A

Action: Required as a cofactor in many biochemical processes.

Uses: Treatment and prophylaxis of vitamin A deficiency.

Dosage:

- Severe deficiency:
  Adults and children > 8 years (PO): 500,000 units/day for 3 days, then 50,000 units/day for 14 days. (IM): 100,000 units/day for 3 days, then 50,000 units/day for 14 days
  Children 1–8 years (PO): 5000 units/kg/day for 5 days, then 5000–10,000 units/day for 2 months. (IM): 15,000–35,000 units/day for 10 days
  Infants (IM): 7500–15,000 units/day followed by PO doses of 5000–10,000 units/day for 10 days
- Prophylaxis: Given every 4–6 months
  Infants ≤ 1 year: 100,000 units. Children > 1 year: 200,000 units.

Brands: 50,000 units Tab; 50,000 units Cap; 50,000 units Inj; Vitamin A.

Side Effects: Seen with overdoses raised ICP, jaundice, vomiting, intracranial hypertension.

Nursing Considerations:

- **Assess:** Monitor patient receiving > 25,000 units/day, as these doses are associated with toxicity. Signs and symptoms of deficiency (growth, night blindness, drying of cornea, dry brittle nails, hair loss, urinary straining, infection)
- **Administration:** Per oral with food
- **Desired Outcome:** Improvement in signs and symptoms of deficiency

2. Vitamin D Compounds

Action: Vitamin D promotes the absorption of calcium and decreases parathyroid hormone concentration.

Uses: Calcitriol; management of hypocalcemia in CRF, treatment of hypocalcemia in hypoparathyroidism, vitamin D resistant and dependent rickets. Vitamin D_3/alfacalcidol; rickets and osteomalacia.

Dosage: (a) Calcitriol

- Management of hypocalcemia in CRF
  Hemodialysis patient:
  IV: Adults: 0.5 mg/kg 3 times/week. Children: 0.01–0.05 mg/kg 3 times/week
  PO: Adults: 0.25 mg. Children; 0.25–2 mg/day
  Nonhemodialysis patient: PO
  Adults and children > 3 years: 0.25 mg/day
  Children < 3 years: 0.01–0.015 mg/kg once daily
- Hypothyroidism:
  Adults and children > 6 years: 0.5–2 mg OD
  Children 1–5 years: 0.25–0.75 mg OD
  Children < 1 year: 0.04–0.08 mg OD
- Vitamin D dependent rickets: PO
  Adults and children: 1 mg OD
- Vitamin D resistant rickets: PO
  Adults and children: 0.02–0.06 mg/kg OD.

(b) Vitamin D_3

- Adults (PO): 400–1000 units OD
- Children: Deficiency state; 6,00,000 IU single dose IM. If no healing seen then repeat after 1 month. Maintenance; 400 IU/day PO.

Brands: Calcitriol: 0.25 mg calcitriol + Zn + calcium, Tab; Mintcal. 0.25 mg Cap; Calosto, Caltrol. 1 mg/mL Inj; Calcibest.

Vitamin D_3: 60,000 IU/sachet; Calcirol granules. 3 and 6 lakh IU/ml Inj; Arachitol.

Side Effects: Common side effects are; dizziness, GI disturbances, dyspnea. Serious side effects include; pancreatitis and convulsions.

Nursing Considerations:

- **Assess:** Vitamin D levels, serum calcium, phosphate levels, PTH level, alkaline phosphatase; height, weight, bone pain, weakness, signs of hypocalcemia (paresthesia, muscle twitching, colic, laryngospasm)
- **Administration:** PO±food. IV slowly
- **Desired Outcome:** Improvement in symptoms, resolution of vitamin D deficiency and normalization of serum calcuim and PTH level.

3. Vitamin E/Alpha Tocopherol

Action: Antioxidant, protects RBC membranes against hemolysis in low birth weight neonates.

Uses: Prevention and treatment of deficiency.

Dosage: PO±food.

- Deficiency:
  Adults: 60–75 units/day. Children: 1 unit/kg/day for 2 months
  Neonates: 25–50 units/day for 1 week
- Prevention of Retinopathy of Prematurity (ROP) or Bronchopulmonary Dysplasia (BPD): Neonates and infants: 15–30 units/kg.

Brands: 200, 400 mg Cap; Evion, Evit.

Side Effects: Seen with prolonged large doses. Common side effects are; headache, weakness, blurred vision, gonadal dysfunction. Serious one is Necrotising Enterocolitis (NEC).

Nursing Considerations:

- **Assess:** Serum cholesterol, triglycerides level, signs of vitamin E deficiency (adults and children—anemia, muscle weakness. Neonates—hemolytic anemia, edema, irritability)
- **Desired Outcome:** Decrease in signs and symptoms of vitamin E deficiency.

4. Vitamin K

Action: Cofactor in the hepatic synthesis of factor II, VII, IX, X.

Uses: Prevention and treatment of Hemorrhagic Disease of Newborn (HDN), anticoagulant induced or vitamin K deficiency hypoprothrombinemia.

Dosage: Phytonadione and menadione is discussed. Former is more effective.

(a) Phytonadione:

- HDN (IM): Prevention; 0.5–1 mg within 1 hour after birth
  Treatment: 1–2 mg/day
- Hypoprothrombinemia:
  Due to vitamin K deficiency: Adults (IM, IV): 10 mg. Children > 1 month (IM, IV): 1–2 mg
  Total parenteral nutrition: Adults (IM): 5–10 mg once weekly
  Children (IM, IV): 2–5 mg once weekly

- Oral anticoagulant overdose: Adults (IV): 2.5–10 mg/dose
  Children > 1 month (IV): 0.5–5 mg.

(b) Menadione
Adults (PO): 2–10 mg (menadione)
Adults (PO, IM, IV): 5–15 mg (menadione sodium).

Brands:
- Phytonadione: 1 mg/0.5 mL, 10 mg/mL Inj; 10 mg Tab; kenadion
- Menadione: 5 mg Tab; 10 mg/mL Inj; Stypindon.

Side Effects: GI disturbances, flushing, hemolytic anemia, hyperbilirubinemia.

Nursing Considerations:
- **Assess:** BP, pulse, PT, watch for internal and external bleeding
- **Administration:** PO±food. For IV use dilute in NS/D_3W/DNS and administer at the rate of 1 mg/min
- **Advise:** Avoid IM injection, injury prone activities. Use soft toothbrush, avoid electric razor until coagulation defect is corrected
- **Desired Outcome:** Decreased bleeding, prevention of HDN.

(B) WATER-SOLUBLE VITAMINS

Include:
1. Ascorbic Acid
2. Cyanocobalamin
3. Folic Acid
4. Niacin
5. Pyridoxine
6. Riboflavin
7. Thiamine

For general nursing consideration of each drug refer to main discussion (Page no. 184).

1. Ascorbic Acid/Vitamin C

Action: Necessary for collagen formation and tissue repair.

Uses: Prevention and treatment of scurvy.

Dosage:
- Adults: Treatment (PO, IM): 100–500 mg/day for 14 days
  Prevention (PO): 50–100 mg/day
- Children: Treatment (PO, IM): 100–300 mg/day for 14 days
  Prevention (PO): 30–45 mg/day.

Brands: 200 mg Tab; Vitamin C, Celin, Limcee. 100 mg/mL Inj; Tildoxon.

Side Effects: Flushing, headache, diarrhea, nausea, vomiting, hemorrhage in patients with G6PD deficiency.

Nursing Consideration: PO ± food. For prophylaxis use either PO or IM and for treatment prefer only PO.

2. Cyanocobalamin

Refer hematinics (Chapter 34).

3. Folic Acid

Refer hematinics (Chapter 34).

4. Niacin/Vitamin B_3

Action: Decreased lipolysis, increased lipoprotein lipase and decreased esterification of triglycerides.

Uses: Treatment and prevention of Pellagra, adjunctive therapy in certain hyperlipidemias.

Dosage: PO+food to decrease GI discomfort.

- Adults and children: Deficiency: 200–500 mg/day in divided doses
- Hyperlipidemias: 100–500 mg/day (Max: 10 mg/kg/day)
- Children 4–10 years: 12 mg/day
- Birth 3 years: 5–9 mg/day.

Brands: 375, 500 mg Tab; Neasyn - SR, Nialip.

Side Effects: Common side effects are; GI upset, upper body flushing, pruritus, headache. Serious one is hepatotoxicity.

Nursing Considerations:

- **Assess:** LFT, blood glucose, uric acid, serum cholesterol, triglycerides, cardiac status, signs of deficiency (stomatitis, glossitis, anemia, dermatitis, confusion, delirium)
- **Administration:** Upper body flushing can be decreased by pretreatment with NSAIDs (aspirin) given 30-60 minutes prior to drug. Concurrent intake of hot drinks or alcohol may increase flushing and pruritis
- **Advise:** When using for hyperlipidemias, should be used in conjunction with dietary restriction, smoking cessation and exercise
- **Desired Outcome:** Decrease in signs and symptoms of deficiency. Decrease in serum cholesterol and triglycerides levels.

5. Pyridoxine/Vitamin B_6

Action: Required for amino acids, lipids and carbohydrate metabolism.

Uses: Treatment and prevention of deficiency, treatment of pyridoxine dependent seizures in infants, drug induced neuropathy.

Dosage:

- Treatment of deficiency (PO)
  Adults: 2.5–10 mg/day until clinical signs are corrected then 2.5 mg/day
  Children: 5–25 mg/day for 3 weeks, then 1.5–2.5 mg/day
- Pyridoxine dependent seizures (PO, IM, IV)
  Neonates and infants: Initially 10–100 mg/day parenteral, then 50–100 mg/day orally
- Drug induced neuritis (PO)
  Adults (PO): Treatment: 100–300 mg/day
  Prophylaxis: 25–100 mg/day
  Children(PO): Treatment: 10–50 mg/day
  Prophylaxis: 1–2 mg/kg/day.

Brands: 40 mg Tab; Benadon. 100 mg Tab; B-long.

Side Effects: They are seen with overdoses only. They being sensory neuropathy, paresthesia, flushing.

Nursing Considerations:

- **Assess:** Seizures precautions, signs of deficiency (anemia, nausea, vomiting, seizures, dermatitis, cheilosis)
- **Administration:** PO ± food. Parenterally should only be used if per oral is not possible. Give IV slowly over 30 minutes and monitor pulse, BP and respiration
- **Desired Outcome:** Decrease in the symptoms of deficiency.

6. Riboflavin

Action: Acts as a coenzyme.

Use: Treatment and prevention of deficiency.

Dosage: PO±food. Deficiency: Adults; 5–10 mg/day and children 3–10 mg/day in divided doses.

Brands: 20 mg Tab; Lipabol.

7. Thiamine/Vitamin B_1

Action: Essential coenzyme for carbohydrate metabolism.

Uses: Treatment of beriberi and prevention of Wernicke's encephalopathy.

Dosage:
- Beriberi: Adults (PO): 5–10 mg 3 times/day. (IM, IV): 5–100 mg 3 times/day Children (PO): 10–50 mg/day in divided doses. (IM, IV): 10–25 mg/day in divided doses
- Wernicke's encephalopathy: Adults: Initially 100 mg IV, then 50–100 mg/day IM or IV.

Brands: 75 mg Tab; Benalgis.

Side Effects: Common side effects are; nausea, diarrhea. Serious side effects are; angioedema, vascular collapse.

Nursing Considerations:

- **Assess:** BP, pulse, signs and symptoms of deficiency (GI discomfort, irritability, palpitation, tachycardia, edema, paresthesia, confusion, memory loss, anorexia, muscle weakness, psychosis)
- **Administration:** PO±food. Prefer PO over parenteral usage. Give IV slowly over 5–10 minutes
- **Advise:** Psychosis and confusion takes longer time to respond as compared to other signs and symptoms
- **Desired Outcome:** Decrease in signs of deficiency.

Chapter 47

Miscellaneous

Include: 1. Albumin 2. Rho(D) Immunoglobulin

1. Albumin

Action: Increases intravascular oncotic pressure and causes mobilization of fluid from interstitial to intravascular space.

Uses: Treatment of hypovolemia, plasma volume expansion and maintenance of cardiac output in the treatment of shock, burn, hemorrhage; hypoproteinemia resulting in generalized edema or decreased intravascular volume (nephrotic syndrome, end stage renal disease).

Dosage:

- Hypoproteinemia (IV): Use 25% albumin
  Adults: 50–75 g. Children, infants and neonates: 0.5–1 g/kg/dose may repeat every 1–2 days
- Nephrotic syndrome (IV): Use 25% albumin
  Adults: 12.5–50 g/day in 3–4 divided doses. Children and infants: 0.25–1 g/kg/dose
- Hypovolemic shock (IV): Use 5% albumin
  Adults: 25 g, may repeat as needed. Infants: 0.25–0.5 g/kg/dose.

Brands: 5% albumin in 250 and 500 mL bottle; Albutein, Human albumin. 25% albumin in 50 and 100 mL bottle; Albudac, Human albumin. 20% albumin in 50 and 100 mL bottle; Albudac, Human albumin.

Side Effects: Common side effects are; nausea, vomiting, headache, fluid overload, hypertension, tachycardia, fever, chills. Serious one is pulmonary edema.

Nursing Consideration:

- **Assess:** BP, pulse, respiration, CBC, serum electrolytes and sodium, input and output, signs of hypervolemia, cardiac failure and pulmonary edema
- **Administration:** Administer via large gauge needle. Too rapid infusion may result in vascular overload. Solution should be clear amber, discard discolored or particulate containing solution, use within 4 hours of opening. For hypovolemia infuse over 30–60 minutes and for hypoproteinemia infuse over 2–4 hours at the rate of 2–3 mL/min. It should not be given to burn patients in first 24 hours. 5% is given at the rate of 2–4 mL/min and 25% at 1 mL/min rate
- **Desired Outcome:** Increase in BP, blood volume, urine output and serum plasma proteins.

2. Rho (D) Immunoglobulin

Action: Prevents production of anti-Rho (D) antibodies in Rho (D) negative patients who were exposed to Rho (D) positive blood. Increases platelet count in patients with ITP.

Uses: Suppression of Rh isoimmunization: Used when the mother is Rho (D) negative; father of the child is either Rho (D) positive or unknown; the baby is either Rho (D) positive or unknown. It is used in the following situations; during delivery of an Rho (D) positive infant, abortion, amniocentesis, transplacental hemorrhage.

Treatment of ITP: Used in nonsplenectomized Rho (D) positive individuals.

Dosage: IM

- Pregnancy: Adults: 300 μg at 28 weeks and following delivery within 72 hours
- Postpartum: Adults: 300 μg within 72 hours of delivery
- Abortion, miscarriage, termination of pregnancy: Adults: < 13 weeks gestation: 100 μg. ≥ 13 weeks gestation: 300 μg within 72 hours
- ITP: Adults and children: Initially if Hb ≥ 10 g%; 50 μg/kg as a single dose. If Hb < 10 g%, 25–40 μg/kg as a single dose. Maintenance dose varies (25–60 μg/kg).

Brands: 300 μg/vial; Gynae-D, Rhesuman, Rhogam.

Side Effects: Common side effects are; nausea, vomiting, diarrhea, headache, hypertension, rash, anemia, fever, arthralgia.

Nursing Consideration:

- **Assess:** BP, pulse, respiration, CBC, RFT, platelet and reticulocyte counts, Rho (D) typing of mother and infant; signs and symptoms of intravascular hemolysis
- **Administration:** Use IM into deltoid muscle, do not give into gluteal muscle. Reconstitute with 1.25 mL of NS by injecting diluent onto inside wall of vial and gently shaking until dissolves. Do not shake vial
- **Advise:** Explain to patient that the purpose of this medication is to protect future Rho (D) positive infants
- **Desired Outcome:** Prevention of erythroblastosis fetalis in future Rho (D) positive infants. Decreased bleeding episodes in patients with ITP.

Section 2

Calculation of Drug Dosages

Nurses should know how to calculate drug dosages accurately which is a very important part of their practice. Learning calculation of drug dosage will help them solve dosages problem easily and will build-up their confidence for administering drug safely. For calculating dosages the nurses need to learn some basic mathematics concept of calculation, calculating pediatric dosages, drip rate and maintenance fluid calculation, weight and measures, and in the last, questions with answers explained.

Chapter

48 Learning Basic Mathematics

Whole numbers: Represent amount or quantity of something.

For example, 1 apple — 1 is a whole number

2 tablets — 2 is a whole number

Fraction: Represents a part of a whole number.

For example, 1/2 apple or $\frac{1}{2}$ (1 divided by 2)

or — in a fraction is a division sign.

Parts of fraction : Has two parts.

For example, $\frac{1}{2}$, 1 is a numerator and 2 is a denominator.

Types of fraction:

- Proper fraction: Numerator is smaller than denominator.

  For example, $\frac{1}{2}$ or $\frac{2}{3}$ or $\frac{3}{4}$
- Improper fraction: Numerator is greater than denominator.

  For example, $\frac{2}{1}$ or $\frac{3}{2}$ or $\frac{4}{3}$
- Equal fraction: Numerator and denominator are equal.

  For example, $\frac{1}{1}$ or $\frac{2}{2}$ or $\frac{3}{3}$

Reducing fraction: Always reduce fraction to the lowest term. To reduce, divide numerator and denominator by the same number.

- Reducing proper fraction: For example, $\frac{2}{4}=\frac{2}{4}+\frac{2}{2}=\frac{1}{2}$
- Reducing improper fraction: For example, $\frac{17}{5}$

Divide the numerator by denominator $\frac{17}{5}$= 3 (remainder = 2). 3 becomes the whole number and the remainder is the new numerator, the denominator remains the same, i.e. . $\frac{17}{5}=3\frac{2}{5}$

- Reducing equal fractions: For example, $\frac{4}{4}=\frac{4}{4}+\frac{2}{2}=\frac{2}{2}\div\frac{2}{2}=\frac{1}{1}$

Mixed number: Contains both whole number and fraction.

For example, $1\frac{1}{2}$ (1 is a whole number and $\frac{1}{2}$ is a fraction). Always change the mixed number to improper fraction before solving problems.

For example, $4\frac{1}{8}$, multiply denominator by the whole number, i.e. 4×8 = 32

Add the numerator, the above multiplicate, i.e. 1 + 32 = 33.

Now 33 becomes the new numerator and denominator remains the same.

i.e $=4\frac{1}{8}=\frac{33}{8}$

Lowest common denominator: Fractions can easily be subtracted or added if they have a common denominator. Fractions with different denominators need to have a common denominator before they can be added or subtracted.

- Fraction with common denominators:

Addition: $\frac{1}{5}+\frac{3}{5}=\frac{4}{5}$

Subtraction: $\frac{10}{8}-\frac{7}{8}=\frac{3}{8}$

- Fraction with different denominators:

Addition: $\frac{1}{12}+\frac{3}{4}=\frac{4+36}{48}=\frac{40}{48}=\frac{10}{12}=\frac{5}{6}$

Subtraction: $\frac{5}{6}-\frac{1}{3}=\frac{15-6}{18}=\frac{9}{18}=\frac{1}{2}$

Addition and Subtraction of Fractions:

- Check the denominator before adding and subtracting fractions
- If denominators are same, add or subtract the numerator. The sum/difference becomes the numerator of the answer and the denominator remains the same.

Addition, e.g. $\frac{2}{5}+\frac{1}{5}=\frac{3}{5}$

Subtraction, e.g. $\frac{10}{6}-\frac{4}{6}=\frac{6}{6}=\frac{1}{1}$

- If denominators are different, first find the lowest common denominator, then add/subtract the numerator. The sum/difference becomes the numerator of the answer and the lowest common denominator is the denominator.

Addition, e.g. $\frac{3}{4}+\frac{2}{5}=\frac{15+8}{20}=\frac{23}{20}=1\frac{3}{20}$

Subtraction, e.g. $\frac{7}{8}-\frac{1}{4}=\frac{7-2}{8}=\frac{5}{8}$

- When adding or subtracting mixed numbers, first change to improper fraction then further steps remain the same as stated above.

Addition, e.g. $1\frac{3}{4}+2\frac{5}{8}=\frac{7}{4}+\frac{21}{8}=\frac{14+21}{8}=\frac{35}{8}=4\frac{3}{8}$

Subtraction, e.g. $4\frac{1}{2}-1\frac{2}{3}=\frac{9}{2}-\frac{5}{3}=\frac{27-10}{6}=\frac{17}{6}=2\frac{5}{6}$

Multiplication of fractions: In multiplication there is no need to find a common denominator, just multiply the numerator and denominator then reduce the answer to the lowest terms. In case of mixed numbers first change to improper fraction.

For example, $\frac{6}{7}\times\frac{2}{5}=\frac{12}{35}$

$6\frac{1}{8}\times 3\frac{2}{3}=\frac{49}{8}\times\frac{11}{3}=\frac{539}{24}=22\frac{11}{24}$

Division of fractions: For division, first invert the second fraction and change the division sign to a multiplication sign, further steps remain the same as in multiplication of fraction.

For example, $\frac{2}{5}\div\frac{2}{8}=\frac{2}{5}\times\frac{8}{2}=\frac{16}{10}=\frac{8}{5}=1\frac{3}{5}$

Ratio: A ratio is a comparison of two numbers and these two numbers are related to each other.

For example, 10 mg drug in each tablet, can be written as 10 mg/1 tablet.
10 mg drug per kg of body weight, can be written as 10 mg/1 kg.

Ratio can be written in 2 ways:

linear ratio, i.e. 1:2 (1 is to 2)

For example, 10 mg per 1 mL = 10 mg:1 mL (10 mg is to 1 mL)

Fractional ratio, i.e. $\frac{1}{2}$ (1 divided by 2)

For example, 10 mg per 1 mL = $\frac{10}{1\,\text{mL}}$ (10 mg divided by 1 mL)

Colon (:) or linear line (–) used in ratio represents the division (÷) of two numbers.

Proportion: Proportion is an equation of two ratios.

It can be written in 2 ways:

Linear proportion 1:2: :2:4 (one is to two as two is to four)

Fractional proportion $\frac{1}{2}=\frac{2}{4}$ (one divided by two equals two divided by four)

Proportion has two parts means (2 and 2) and extremes (1 and 4).

Linear ratio and proportion:

For this we should know the known ratio and the unknown ratio.

For example, Chemist supplied 10 mg tablets. Doctor orders to give 5 mg to patient.

The problem can be set as $\underbrace{\text{10 mg:1 tablet}}_{\text{Known ratio}}::\underbrace{\text{5 mg: } x \text{ tablet}}_{\text{Unknown ratio}}$

Units should be in the same order and match each ratio in proportion.

mg:tablet: :mg:tablet

Then solve problem as follows. Product of mean is equal to the product of extremes

$$10 \times x = 5 \times 1$$

$$x = \frac{5 \times 1}{10} = \frac{5}{10} = \frac{1}{2}$$

Answer is, the patient has to give half tablet.

Fractional ratio and proportion: In this numerator of one fraction is multiplied by the denominator of other fraction and vice versa. We should know known and unknown proportion, e.g. Doctor order is to give 10 mg. Chemist supplied 5 mg tablets. The problem can be set as:

$$\underbrace{\frac{5\text{ mg}}{1\text{ tablet}}}_{\text{Known proportion}} = \underbrace{\frac{10\text{ mg}}{x\text{ tablet}}}_{\text{Unknown proportion}}$$

Units should be in the same order and match.

$$\frac{\text{mg}}{\text{tablet}} = \frac{\text{mg}}{\text{tablet}}$$

Then solve the problem as follows.

$$5 \times x = 10 \times 1$$

$$x = \frac{10 \times 1}{5} = \frac{10}{5} = 2 \text{ tablets}$$

Answer is, patient has to give 2 tablets.

Decimal number:

- Decimal numbers have three parts.
  For example, in 2.5, 2 is a whole number
  (.) is a decimal point and separates whole number from decimal fraction
  .5 is the decimal fraction
- *How to read:* 1.1 One point one
  20.45 Twenty point four five
  5.693 Five point six nine three
- If decimal numbers do not contain whole number then place zero in front of decimal point, e.g .5 = 0.5
- *Greater or lesser:*
  For example, 0.2 is greater than 0.02, which is greater than 0.002
  1.5 is greater than 1.49, which is greater than 1.48
- *Changing decimals into fractions:*

  For example, $0.5 = \frac{5}{10}$, $1.50 = \frac{150}{100}$, $1.555 = \frac{1555}{1000}$

  [Count the number of digits on the right of decimal point and then place same number of zero after writing one]

- *Changing fractions into decimals:*

  For example, $\frac{1}{4} = 0.25$, $\frac{1}{2} = 0.5$

- *Addition of decimals:* Line up correctly then add. Decimal point should be in line.

  For example, 132.08 + 82.032 + 1.01

$$\begin{array}{r} 132.08 \\ 82.032 \\ +\quad 1.01 \\ \hline 215.122 \end{array}$$

- *Subtraction of decimals:* Line up correctly then subtract.

  For example, 110.3 - 1.2

$$\begin{array}{r} 110.3 \\ -\quad 1.2 \\ \hline 109.1 \end{array}$$

- *Multiplication of decimals:* Multiply the number without thinking of the decimal place. Then count the total number of places at the right of the decimal point. Then count the same number of places in the answer and place the decimal point.

  For example, $1.5 \times 10 = 15 \times 10 = 150 = 15.0 = 15$

  $2.5 \times 0.5 = 25 \times 5 = 125 = 1.25$

- *Division of decimals:*

  For example, $4.2 \div 2 = 2.1$

  $3.1 \div 2 = 1.55$

- *Finding the percentage:*

  For example, 25% of 200 (25% means 25 parts out of 100)

  $= \frac{25}{100} \times 200 = 50$

  30% of 200 $= \frac{30}{100} \times 200 = 60$

  For example, 2 is what percentage of 10 = $\frac{2}{10} \times 100 = 20\%$

  3 is what percentage of 10 = $\frac{3}{10} \times 100 = 30\%$

Chapter 49 Weights and Measures

Sometimes the unit in which the dose is ordered may differ from the unit in which the medicine is available. Doctor may order in milligram but the drug is available in grams or the order is in microgram and the drug is available in grams or the order is in milliliter and the fluid is available in liter or the drug is available in perfilled syrings and the order is in milligram. For these conversion the nursing staff should know the units of measurements, equivalent measurements and abbreviations/symbols used, etc.

Unit		Approximate value
1 kg (kilogram)	=	1000 g (grams)
	=	2.2 lbs (pounds)
1 lbs	=	454 g
1 g	=	1000 mg (milligram)
1 mg	=	1000 µg (microgram)
1 µg	=	0.001 mg
1 L (liter)	=	1000 mL (milliliter)
	=	2 pints
1 mL	=	15 drops/60 microdrops
1 pint	=	500 mL
1 Oz (ounce)	=	30 mL
1 teaspoonful	=	5 mL
1 teacupful	=	150 mL
1 glassful	=	200 mL
1 inch	=	2.54 cm (centimeter)
1 cm	=	10 mm (millimeter)

Chapter

50 Methods of Calculating Drug Dosages

There are various methods of calculation. Learn them accurately and you can use anyone of them according to your convenience.

1. **Linear ratio and proportion method**
2. **Fractional ratio and proportion method**
3. **Formula method:**

(Both these methods are explained in the section of basic mathematics)

$$\frac{\text{Amount ordered}}{\text{Amount in hand}} \times \text{Vehicle} = \text{Number of tablets, capsules or amount of liquid}$$

Vehicle is the drug form or amount of liquid containing the dosage. Amounts used in calculation by formula must be in the same system.

For example, Chemist supplied 100 mg Cefixime tablets. Order is to give 200 mg/dose twice daily.

Ans: Amount ordered is 200 mg. Amount in hand is 100 mg tablets. Vehicle is tablet.

$$\frac{200\,\text{mg}}{100\,\text{mg}} \times \text{tablets} = \frac{2}{1} = 2 \text{ tablets/dose has to be given.}$$

4. **Dimensional analysis method:**

$$\text{Order in mg} \times \frac{\text{1 tablet or capsule}}{\text{that 1 tablet or capsule is in mg}} = \text{Tablets or capsules to be given}$$

Amounts used in calculation of formula must be in the same system.

For example: Chemist supplied 250 mg Amoxycillin capsules. Order is to give 500 mg/dose.

Ans: Order is 500 mg. 1 Capsule is 250 mg.

$$500\text{ mg} \times \frac{\text{Capsule}}{250\text{ mg}} = 2 \text{ capsule/dose has to be given.}$$

Chapter

51 Calculating Pediatric Drug Dosages

For calculating dosage in children nurses must know child's weight in kg or the Body Surface Area (BSA) and the recommended formulary doses. Pediatric dosages are recommended as mg/kg/dose or mg/kg/day or $\mu g/m^2$/dose or $\mu g/m^2$/day. Various formulas are also available to calculate pediatric doses from the known adult dosage.

1. **Friends formula** (for children < 1 year of age).

$$\frac{\text{Age of the child in months}}{150} \times \text{Adult's dose} = \text{Child's dose}$$

For example, if the adult dose of a drug is 500 mg/dose, calculate the amount of drug/dose for an infant of 6 months age.

Ans: $\frac{6\,\text{months}}{150} \times 500 = \frac{2}{5} \times 50 = 20$ mg/dose.

2. **Young formula** (for children > 1 years of age upto 12 years).

$$\frac{\text{Age of the child in years}}{\text{Age of the child in years} + 12} \times \text{Adult's dose} = \text{Child's dose}$$

For example, if the adult dose of a drug is 500 mg/dose, calculate the amount of drug for a child aged 6 years.

Ans: $\frac{6\,\text{years}}{6+12} \times 500 = \frac{6}{18} \times 500 = 166$ mg/dose.

3. **Clark's formula** (can be used for children of all ages).

$$\frac{\text{Weight of the child in pounds}}{150} \times \text{Adult's dose} = \text{Child's dose}$$

For example, if the adult dose of a drug is 250/day, calculate the dose for a child weighing 30 pounds.

Ans: $\frac{30\,\text{Pounds}}{150} \times 250 = \frac{3}{15} \times 250 = \frac{1}{5} \times 250 = 50$ mg/dose.

4. **Body surface area (BSA) method.**

$$\frac{\text{BSA}}{1.7} \times \text{Adult's dose} = \text{Child's dose}$$

For example, if the adult dose of a drug is 200 mg/day, calculate the dose for a child with BSA of 0.34 m^2.

Ans: $\frac{0.34}{1.7} \times 200 = 40 \text{ mg/day}$.

Chapter

52 Calculating Maintenance Fluid Requirements in Children

Pediatric patients once fall ill stop taking orally or do not take anything orally enough. Then they have to be either admitted or put on day care treatment and to prevent dehydration they have to be given maintenance fluids. There are two methods available to calculate maintenance fluid requirement.

A. **Body weight method:** For this child's weight in kg should be known.
< 10 kg = 100 mL/kg
11–20 kg = 1000 mL + 50 mL/kg for each kg > 10
> 20 kg = 1500 mL + 20 mL/kg for each kg > 20
For example, calculate maintenance fluid for child weighing 24 kg.
Ans: For first 10 kg = 1000 mL (10×100 mL)
For second 10 kg = 500 mL (10×50 mL)
For 4 kg (>20 kg) = 80 mL (4×20 mL)
Total = 1000 + 500 + 80 = 1580 mL is the maintenance fluid for the child/day.

$$\text{Fluid rate} = \frac{1580 \text{ mL}}{24 \text{ hr}} = 65.83 \text{ mL/hr} = 66 \text{ mL/hr (after rounding of)}$$

B. **Body surface area (BSA) method:** For this child's BSA should be known.
This method is commonly used in children >10 kg.
Range is 1500 to 2000 mL/m^2/day
Formula:
1500–2000 mL/m^2/day ÷ 24 = fluid rate in mL/hr
For example, calculate fluid rate in mL/hr for a child with BSA of 0.6 m^2
Ans: 1500 mL/m^2/day × 0.6 m^2 = 900 mL/day ÷ 24 hours = 37.5 mL/hr.
2000 mL/m^2/day × 0.6 m^2 = 1200 mL/day ÷ 24 hours = 50 mL/hr.
Maintenance fluid rate range is 37.5–50 mL/hr.

Chapter

53 IV Drip Rate Calculation

IV fluids are given by two ways either by gravity flow or by pump. If given by gravity flow, to regulate the rate nurses should calculate the flow rate in drops/minute. If giving via infusion pump, the nurses should calculate mL/hr of infusion.

To calculate the drip rate following information is needed:

- Amount of solution to be given (volume)
- Duration for which it has to be given (hour or minutes)
- Drop factor of IV tubing.

For example, Doctor orders to give 800 mL of normal saline (NS) over 4 hours.

Ans: Volume is 800 mL (or 800 mL/4 hr = 200 mL/hr), duration is 4 hours and drop factor can be found out on IV tube label.

$$\frac{\text{Volume}}{\text{Duration}} = \text{mL/hr or minutes}$$

To convert hours to minutes: 1 hour = 60 minutes

To convert mL to drop: 15 drops = 1 mL

Set-up each of the values in a proportion.

$$\frac{200\,\text{mL}}{1\text{hr}} \times \frac{1\text{hr}}{60\,\text{min}} \times \frac{15\,\text{drops}}{1\text{mL}}$$

Cancel number and units of measure from upper and lower level of the equation.

$$\frac{200 \times 15\text{ drops}}{60\text{ min}} = \frac{300\,\text{drops}}{60\,\text{min}} = \frac{50\text{ drops}}{\text{min}}$$

So, the infusion rate is 200 mL/hr or 50 drops/min.

Chapter

54 Administering Medicines to Children

Medication administration to pediatric population is a very difficult job. One child may take the particular product and form of medicine easily but the another child may not accept the same.

Nurses should learn following points for administering medicines to children:

- In children oral route is preferred over parenteral. If not accepting one type of oral form, try another form
- Special equipments are available for administering oral medicines, e.g. measuring cups and spoons, oral syringes, oral droppers, cylindrical dosing spoons. Parents should be taught to use caliberated devices provided with product rather than using household utensils
- In young children, it is better to give part of the dose at a time into the side of the cheek away from the bitter taste buds at the back of the tongue
- Prefer liquid preparation in children <5 years of age and in >5 years of age give dispersible or chewable form of medicines
- Maximum volume allowed in parenteral administration is; subcutaneous = 0.5, intradermal = 0.01–0.1 mL, intramuscular 0.5–1 mL, intravenous = use smallest recommended diluent for dilution
- For IM prefer shorter (0.5–1 inch) and smaller (23–30 Gauge) needles
- Give IV via pediatric drip set with microdrip chamber
- For ID route use 1 mL syringes caliberated in 0.01 mL units and 26–27 Gauge needles
- For SC route use 1 mL syringe caliberated in 40 or 80 units and 25 Gauge needles
- Always compare the ordered dose with the recommended formulary dose based on a child's weight or Body Surface Area (BSA). Ordered dose is considered safe if it is less than or equal to the recommended formulary dose.

Chapter

55 Solving Problems

This chapter contains some practical problems related to dose calculation, to be solved by the nurses knowledge gained in the previous sections shall be used to some these.
Few problems are set-up for solving by the nurses. Use your knowledge explained and learned in the previous sections. Use calculator if required.

1. Doctor order is for 125 mg azithromycin/day. Chemist sends 250 mg tablets. How many tablets nurse has to give?

Ans: Using linear ratio and proportion method.

Known ratio = 250 mg : 1 tablet

Unknown ratio = 125 mg : x tablet

$$\Rightarrow 250:1::125:x = 250\,x = 125 \;\Rightarrow x = \frac{125}{250} = \frac{1}{2}$$

Nurse has to give ½ tablet.

2. Doctor order is for 75 mg cefpodoxime. Chemist gives 50 mg tablets. How many tablets will the nurse give?

Ans: Using fractional ratio and proportion method.

Known ratio = 50 mg: 1 tablet

Unknown ratio = 75 mg: x tablets

$$\Rightarrow \frac{50\,\text{mg}}{1\,\text{tablet}} = \frac{75}{x} \;\Rightarrow 50x = 75 \times 1 \;\Rightarrow x = \frac{75}{50} = 1.5\,\text{tablets}$$

Nurse has to give $1\frac{1}{2}$ tablets.

3. Chemist sends 0.25 mg alprazolam tablets. Order is for 0.5 mg. How many tablets will the nurse give?

Ans: Using formula method: $\frac{\text{Desired dose}}{\text{Dose in hand}} \times \text{Vehicle} = \text{x Tablet/Capsule}$

Desired dose = 0.5 mg. Dose in hand = 0.25 mg. Vehicle = tablet

$$\frac{0.5\,\text{mg}}{0.25\,\text{mg}} \times \text{tablet} = \frac{5}{2.5} = 2\,\text{tablets}$$

Nurse has to give 2 tablets.

4. Doctor order is for 25 mg Cefixime. Chemist sends 50 mg/5 mL syrup. How many mL will the nurse give?

Ans: Using linear ratio and proportion method:

Known ratio = 50 mg : 5 mL Unknown ratio = 25 mg : x

50 mg : 5 mL :: 25 mg : x

$$50x = 5 \times 25 \Rightarrow x = \frac{125}{50} \Rightarrow \frac{25}{10} = 2.5\,\text{mL}$$

Nurse has to give 2.5 mL of the syrup.

5. Doctor order is for 4 mg ondensetron IV. Chemist sends 2 mg/mL vial. How many mL will the nurse give?

Ans: Using fractional ratio and proportion method:

Known ratio = 2 mg: 1 mL Unknown ratio = 4 mg:x mL

$$\frac{2\,\text{mg}}{1\,\text{mL}} = \frac{4\,\text{mg}}{x\,\text{mL}}$$

$$2x = 4 \times 1 \Rightarrow x = \frac{4}{2} = 2\,\text{ml}$$

Nurse has to give 2 ml.

6. Order is for 100 mg/day of colistin sulfate. Pharmacy sends 12.5 mg/5 mL syrup. How many mL will nurse give?

Ans: Using formula method: $\frac{\text{Desired dose}}{\text{Dose in hand}} \times \text{Vehicle}$

Desired dose = 100 mg. Dose in hand = 12.5 mg. Vehicle = 5 mL Syrup.

$$\frac{100\,\text{mg}}{12.5\,\text{mg}} \times 5\,\text{mL Syrup} \Rightarrow \frac{1000}{125} \times 5 \Rightarrow \frac{1000}{25} = 40\,\text{mL Syrup}$$

Nurse has to give 40 mL syrup per day.

7. Doctor orders 25 μg levothyroxine/day once daily. Chemist sends a bottle of 30 tablets, each tablet contains 50 μg. How many days will this bottle last?

Ans: Using fractional ratio and proportion method:

Known ratio = 50 μg: 1 tablet. Unknown ratio = 25 μg: x

$$\frac{50\,\mu\text{g}}{1\,\text{tablet}} = \frac{25\,\mu\text{g}}{x} \Rightarrow x = \frac{25 \times 1}{50} \Rightarrow x = \frac{1}{2}\,\text{tablet}$$

Half tablet has to be given per day. Therefore 30 tablets will last for 60 days.

$$\left\{ \frac{0.5\,\text{tablet}}{1\,\text{day}} = \frac{30\,\text{tablets}}{x} \Rightarrow x = \frac{30 \times 1}{0.5} \Rightarrow \frac{300}{5} = 60\,\text{days} \right\}$$

8. Doctor order is 150 mg amikacin IV twice daily. Chemist sends a vial labelled as 250 mg/mL. How much the patient will receive?

Ans: Using fractional ratio and proportion method:

$$\text{Known ratio} = \frac{250\,\text{mg}}{1\,\text{mL}} \qquad \text{Unknown ratio} = \frac{150\,\text{mg}}{\text{x}\,\text{mL}}$$

$$\frac{250\,\text{mg}}{1\,\text{mL}} = \frac{150\,\text{mg}}{\text{x}\,\text{mL}} \Rightarrow x = \frac{150 \times 1}{250} \Rightarrow \frac{15}{25} \Rightarrow \frac{3}{5} = 0.6\,\text{mL}$$

Patient will receive 0.6 mL/dose twice daily.

9. Doctor order is for 75 mg cefpodoxime twice daily. Chemist sends a bottle labelling 50 mg/5 mL, 60 mL bottle. How many days will the bottle last?

Ans: Formula method: $\frac{\text{Desired dose}}{\text{Dose in hand}} \times \text{Vehicle} = x\,\text{mL Syrup}$

$$\frac{75\,\text{mg}}{50\,\text{mg}} \times 5\,\text{mL Syrup} \Rightarrow \frac{3}{2} \times 5 \Rightarrow \frac{15}{2} \Rightarrow 7.5\,\text{mL}$$

Dose is 7.5 mL/dose. It is to be given twice daily, i.e. 15 mL/day (7.5 × 2 = 15 mL). Therefore 60 mL bottle will last for 4 days (15 × 4 = 60 mL).

10. Doctor order is for 650 mg cefotaxime thrice daily. How many gram dose the patient receive per dose?

Ans: 1000 mg = 1g (using conversion).

$$\therefore 650\,\text{mg} = \frac{1}{1000} \times 650 = \frac{65}{100} = 0.65\,\text{g}$$

Patient will receive 0.65 g/dose.

11. Physician order is for 0.5 mg midazolam. Chemist supplied 5 mg/mL ampule. How many mL will the patient receive?

Ans: Using linear ratio and proportion method.

Known ratio = 5 mg : 1 mL   Unknown ratio = 0.5 mg : x mL.

5 mg : 1 mL :: 0.5 mg : x mL

5x = 0.5 × 1

$$x = \frac{0.5}{5} = \frac{5}{50} = \frac{1}{10} = 0.1\,\text{mL}$$

Patient will receive 0.1 mL.

12. Doctor order is for 0.1 mg levothyroxine per day. Pharmacy sends 50 μg tablets. How may tablets will the patient receive?

Ans: Available and ordered units are different. Therefore first convert anyone of them. Converting ordered dose.

1 mg = 1000 μg.

$$\therefore\ 0.1\,\text{mg} = \frac{1000}{1} \times 0.1 = \frac{1000 \times 1}{10} = 100\,\mu\text{g}\ (\text{dose to be given i.e. 2 tablets})$$

Using fractional ratio and proportion method.

$$\text{Known ratio} = \frac{50\,\mu\text{g}}{1\,\text{tablet}} \quad \text{Unknown ratio} = \frac{100\,\mu\text{g}}{x}$$

$$\frac{50\,\mu\text{g}}{1\,\text{tablet}} = \frac{100\,\mu\text{g}}{x} \Rightarrow 50x = 100 \times 1 \Rightarrow x = \frac{100}{50} = 2\,\text{tablets}$$

Patient will receive 2 tablets per day.

13. Doctor order is to give 20 mEq of KCl/day diluted in water. Chemist sends a 30 mEq/15 mL bottle. How many mL will the patient receive?

Ans: Using formula method: $\frac{\text{Ordered dose}}{\text{Dose in hand}} \times \text{Vehicle} = \text{mL Syrup}$

$$\frac{20\,\text{mEq}}{30\,\text{mEq}} \times 15\,\text{mL Syp} \Rightarrow \frac{2}{3} \times 15 \Rightarrow \frac{30}{3} = 10\,\text{mL Syrup}$$

Patient will receive 10 mL/day of KCl.

14. Order is for 3 teaspoonsfull (tsf) of antacid. How many mL the patient will receive?

Ans: 1 tsf = 5 mL
3 tsf = 5 × 3
= 15 mL
Patient will receive 15 mL of antacid.

15. Doctor order is for 0.25 mg of digoxin syrup. How many μg will the patient receive?

Ans: 1 mg = 1000 μg.

$$\therefore\; 0.25\,\text{mg} = \frac{1000}{1} \times 0.25 = \frac{1000 \times 25}{100} = 250\,\mu\text{g}$$

Patient will receive 250 μg of digoxin syrup.

16. Doctor order is for 10 g lactulose/day. Chemist supplied 10 g/15 mL syrup. How many teaspoonsfull (tsf) will the patient receive?

Ans: Using fractional ratio and proportion method:

$$\text{Known ratio} = \frac{10\,\text{g}}{15\,\text{mL}} \quad \text{Unknown ratio}\ \frac{10\,\text{g}}{x\,\text{mL}}$$

$$\frac{10\,\text{gm}}{15\,\text{mL}} = \frac{10\,\text{gm}}{x\,\text{mL}} \Rightarrow 10x = 10 \times 15 \Rightarrow x = \frac{150}{10} \Rightarrow x = 15\,\text{mL}$$

Since the ordered dose is in tsf, converting mL into tsf
5 mL = 1 tsf

$$\therefore\; 15\,\text{mL} = \frac{1}{5} \times 15 \Rightarrow \frac{15}{5} \Rightarrow \frac{3}{1} \Rightarrow 3\,\text{tsf}$$

Patient will receive 3 tsf/day of lactulose.

17. Physician order is for 1.5 L fluid per day to a patient. Chemist supplied 500 mL bottles. How many bottles will the nurse give per day?

Ans: Ordered unit and supplied units are different.

Converting order unit:

1 L = 1000 mL

$$\therefore\ 1.5\text{L} = \frac{1000}{1} \times 1.5 = \frac{1000 \times 15}{10} = 1500\ \text{mL (amount to be given)}$$

Using formula method:

$$\frac{\text{Desired dose}}{\text{Dose in hand}} \times \text{Vehicle}$$

Desired dose = 1500 mL, Dose in hand = 500 mL, Vehicle = bottles.

$$\frac{1500\,\text{mL}}{500\,\text{mL}} \times \text{bottles} \Rightarrow \frac{15}{5} \Rightarrow 3\,\text{bottles}$$

Nurse will give 3 bottles/day.

Appendix

1 Practically Useful Charts and Tables

Table 1: Equipment for Resuscitation in Various Age Groups

Equipment	*Premature*	*Newborn*	*6 months*	*1–2 years*	*5 years*	*8–10 years*
Chest tubes	10–14 F	12–18 F	14–20 F	14–24 F	20–32 F	28–38 F
N-G tubes	5 feedings	5–8 feedings	8 F	10 F	10–12 F	14–18 F
Foleys	5 feedings	5–8 feedings	8 F	10 F	10–12 F	12 F
Oxygen masks	Newborn	Newborn	Pediatric	Pediatric	Pediatric	Adult
ET tubes	2.5–3.0	3 to 3.5	3.5–4.5	4.0–4.5	5.0–5.5	5.5–6.5
Arm boards	6 inches	6 inches	6–8 inches	8 inches	8–15 inches	15 inches
BP cuffs	Newborn	Newborn	Infant or Child	Child	Child	Child or Adult
Laryngoscope blade	0	1	1	1	2	Adult

Table 2: Fasting Guidelines for Sedation or Anesthesia

Food	*Hours of Fasting Required*
Clear liquids	2
Breast milk	2–4
Formula or light meal (no fat)	6
Full meal	8

Table 3: Sedation Techniques Suggested for Children

Procedure	*Sedation and Analgesia Technique*
Lumbar puncture	• **Local anesthesia with minimal/moderate** sedation Local anesthetics: Lidocaine/EMLA cream minimal/moderate Sedation: Midazolam or sometimes • **Deep sedation: Fentanyl/Midazolam or Ketamine**
Painful procedures: Biopsy of **Liver/Kidney, Bone marrow** aspiration. Fracture reduction.	Deep sedation combined with local anesthesia: As above
Drainage of abscess, Burn debridement, Laceration repair	Local anesthesia with minimal/moderate/deep sedation: As above
IV catheter placement	Local anesthesia and sometimes minimal/moderate sedation: As above

Table 4: Drip Calculations

Drug	*Dose*	*Calculation*	*Rate and Dose*
Dobutamine	5–20 µg/kg/min	6 × body wt (kg) is the mg added to make 100 mL	1 mL/h = 1 µg/kg/min
Dopamine	2–20 µg/kg/min	6 × body wt (kg) is the mg added to make 100 mL	1mL/h = 1 µg/kg/min
Epinephrine	0.1–1 µg/kg/min	0.6 × body wt (kg) is the mg added to make 100 mL	1 mL/h = 0.1 µg/kg/min
Isoproterenol	0.1–1 µg/kg/min	0.6 × body wt (kg) is the mg added to make 100 mL	1mL/h = 0.1 µg/kg/min
Lidocaine	20–50 µg/kg/min	120 mg in 100 mL of D-5%	1 mL/kg/h = 20 µg/kg/min

- **Patients < 40 kg and those requiring fluid restriction may need more concentrated solutions in order to deliver less fluid per hour. In those cases or as an alternative** to the listed calculations above, use the following equation:

$$\text{Rate (mL/h)} = \frac{\text{dose } (\mu\text{g/kg/min} \times \text{weight (kg)} \times 60 \text{ min/h})}{\text{Concentration } (\mu\text{g/mL})}$$

Table 5: Treatment for Drug Extravasation

Medication Extravasated	*Cold/Warm Pack*	*Treatment*
Ischemic Inducer: Dobutamine Dopamine Epinephrine Norepinephrine Phenyleprine Vasopressin	None	Phentolamine: Mix 5 mg with 9 mL of normal saline (NS). Inject a small amount of this solution into extravasated area. Blanching should reverse immediately. Monitor site, if blanching recurs, additional injections of phentolamine may be needed.
Miscellaneous agents: Aminophylline Calcium salts Dextrose Mannitol Phenytoin Contrast media Sodium bicarbonate Sodium chloride Tetracycline	Cold	Hyaluronidase: Add 1 mL NS to 150 units to make 15 units/mL. Administer 0.2 mL SC or intradermally into the extravasated site.

Table 6: Estimation of Total Body Surface Area of Burn Involvement (% by site and age)

Site	*0–1 year*	*1–4 years*	*5–9 years*	*10–14 years*	*15 years*	*Adults*
Head	9.5	8.5	6.5	5.5	4.5	3.5
Neck	0.5	0.5	0.5	0.5	0.5	0.5
Trunk	13	13	13	13	13	13
Upper arm	2	2	2	2	2	2
Forearm	1.5	1.5	1.5	1.5	1.5	1.5
Hand	1.5	1.5	1.5	1.5	1.5	1.5
Perineum	1	1	1	1	1	1
Buttock	2.5	2.5	2.5	2.5	2.5	2.5
Thigh	2.75	3.25	4	4.25	4.5	4.75
Leg	2.5	2.5	2.75	3.00	3.25	3.5
Foot	1.75	1.75	1.75	1.75	1.75	1.75

1. The total body surface area of burn involvement is determined by the sum of the percentages of each site.
2. Applicable to second and third degree burns.
3. Percentage for each site is only for a single extremity with anterior or posterior involvement. Percentage should be doubled if both anterior and posterior of a single extremity is involved.

Parkland Fluid Replacement Formula

A guideline for replacement of deficits and ongoing losses (Note: For infants, maintenance fluids may need to be added to this). Administer 4 mL/kg/% burn of Ringer's lactate (glucose may be added but beware of stress hyperglycemia) over the first 24 hours; half of this total is given over the first 8 hours calculated from the time of injury; the remaining half is given over the next 16 hours. The second 24 hours fluid requirements averages 50% to 75% of first day's requirements. Concentrations and rates are best determined by monitoring weight, serum electrolytes, urine output, nasogastric (NG) losses, etc.

Colloid may be added after 18–24 hours (1 g/kg/day of albumin) to maintain serum albumin > 2 g/100 mL.

Potassium is generally withheld for the first 48 hours due to the large amount of potassium that is released from damaged tissues. To manage serum electrolytes, monitor urine electrolytes twice weekly and replace calculated urine losses.

Table 7: Average Weight and Surface Area

Age	*Average Weight (kg)*[1]	*Approximate Surface Area (m²)*
Weeks gestation		
26	0.9–1	0.1
30	1.3–1.5	0.12
32	1.6–2	0.15
38	2.9–3	0.2
40 (term infant at birth)	3.1–4	0.25
Months		
3	5	0.29
6	7	0.38
9	8	0.42
Year		
1	10	0.49
2	12	0.55
3	15	0.64
4	17	0.74
5	18	0.76
6	20	0.82
7	23	0.90
8	25	0.95
9	28	1.06
10	33	1.18
11	35	1.23
12	40	1.34
Adult	70	1.73

[1]Weights from age 3 months and over are rounded off to the nearest kilogram.

Table 8: Calculation of Surface Area from Weight

Weight Range	*Surface Area*
1–5 Kg	(0.05 × weight) + 0.05
6–10 Kg	(0.04 × weight) + 0.10
11–20 Kg	(0.04 × weight) + 0.20
21–40 Kg	(0.02 × weight) + 0.40

Table 9: Calorie Values of Common Preparation per Serving

Name	*Weight (g)*	*Household Measures*	*Calories*
Chapati	40	1	140
Bread	20	1	40
Khichdi	120	1 katori	140
Khakra	50	1	130
Paratha	80	1	250
Wheat puri (small)	15	1	50
Rice	120	1 katori	100
Pulao	120	1 katori	200
Moong dal	150	1 katori	100
Egg boiled	30	1	60
Egg omelet	60	1	200
Fish fry	60	1 slice	100
Tea*	150 mL	1 medium cup	20
Coffee*	150 mL	1 medium cup	20
Buttermilk	150 mL	1 medium cup	45
Fruit salad	150	1 serving	150
Ice cream	150	1 slice	380
Rice kheer	150	1 Katori	345
Jalebi	25	1 piece	140
Rasgulla	50	1 piece	150
Samosa	80	1 piece	125
Onion bhajiya	45	6 pieces	150
Idli	20	1 piece	75
Dahiwada	40	1 piece	80
Mango juice*	200 mL	1 glass	150
Orange juice*	200 mL	1 glass	64
Sugarcane juice*	200 mL	1 glass	76
Lime juice*	200 mL	1 glass	60
Potato wafers	50	1 serving	430

*Values are without sugar.

Appendix

2 Methods of Administration of Medications

PRE-REQUISITES

- Ask for any history of allergy/drug reactions
- Understand doctor's orders regarding route of administration, dose to be given etc.
- Medicine to be given should be at the room temperature except the suppositories
- Wash hands with soap and water for 2 minutes using WHO's 6 step technique or alternatively alcohol based waterless antiseptic handrub can be used
- Select the site to be used, clean it with alcohol and let it dry before using the site. Maintain proper asepsis
- Restrain the patient if required
- Wear gloves then load the syringe with the ordered amount of drug and any air should be completely removed from the syringe and needle before injecting
- Dispose syringe and needle immediately after use. Better to use autodisable (AD) syringes. Do not recap the needles
- Injection site should not be rubbed following injection. Apply pressure with cotton after injection to prevent bleeding/back flow of drug
- Do not mix different medicines in single syringe unless recommended
- Always record the name and amount of the drug given.

Mathematics

Knowledge of mathematics will be helpful during injection.

- **Angle:** It is a space between two straight lines that meet

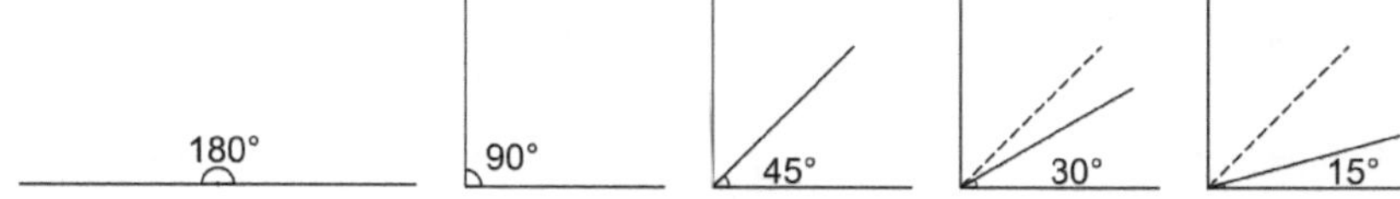

- **Parallel:** Two lines staying at equal distance from each other or maintaining equal distance are called parallel lines.

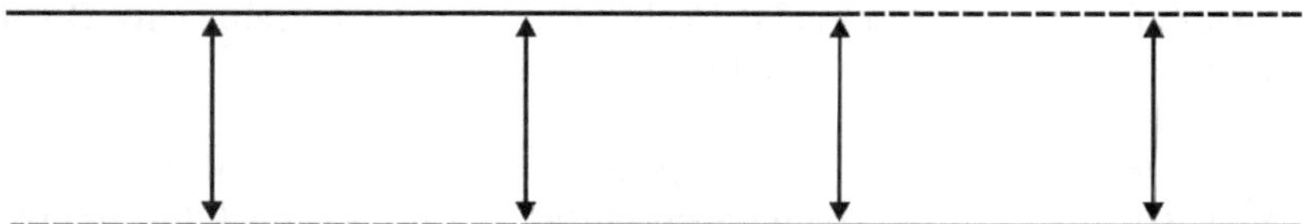

Holding Needle and Syringes

- Needle has two edges, a smooth curved edge and a slanting edge (bevel). The bevel of the needle should always be faced upwards while giving injection

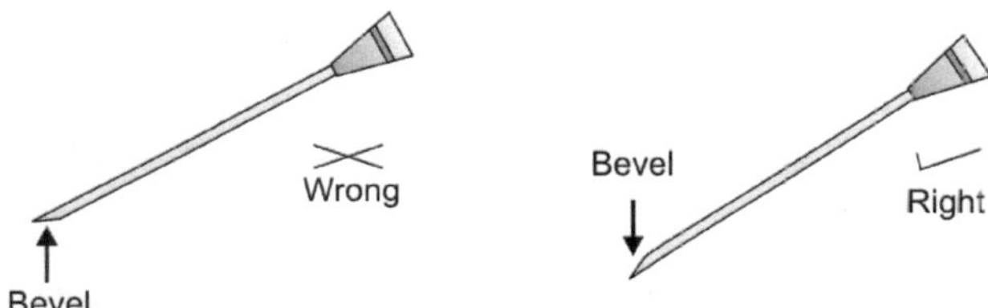

- Syringes may have either central or eccentric nozzle. If holding syringes at an angle of 90° both types can be held in a same way; but if holding at an angles less than 90° always hold in a way shown below.

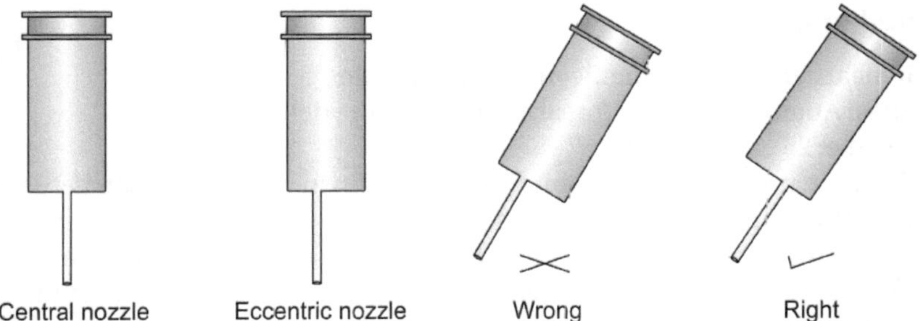

Intramuscular Injection

- It means injection of medicine into the muscle mass
- Sites: Adults: Gluteal, Deltoid, Vastus, Triceps etc.
  Pediatric : <2 years and in malnourished children; Vastus
  : >2 years; Vastus, Gluteal, Deltoid
- Needle: 23–25 gauge
- Enter the needle into the muscle, keeping an angle of 45°–90° with the skin, after reaching the muscle and before injecting drug pull back the plunger to confirm that no blood is seen in the syringe, then only push the medicine. Wait for a few seconds, then pull back slowly and apply pressure using sterile cotton to prevent oozing of blood and back flow of drug.

Intravenous Injection

- It means injection of medicine directly into the venous system
- Sites: Cubital fossa, Antibracheal Veins, Dorsalis pedis, Scalp veins, Great saphenous vein, interdigital veins, Jugular veins etc.
- Needle: 23–25 gauge
- Enter the needle into the vein keeping an angle of 15°–30° with the skin. After reaching the vein (blood seen in the needle) pull back the syringe plunger to see blood is flowing freely, then only slowly push the medicine. Wait for few seconds, pull back the needle and apply pressure with a cotton swab to prevent bleeding and back flow of drug
- If frequent IV administration is required then it is better to fix a intravenous catheter.

Subcutaneous Injection

- It means injection of medicine beneath the skin
- Site: Area around the umbilicus, Anterolateral aspect of thigh, Posterior aspect of arm
- Needle: 23–25 gauge
- Enter the needle into the subcutaneous space keeping an angle of 45° with the skin and draw back the plunger to make sure there is no blood, then slowly push the medicine. A proper injection will cause a round wheal at the injection site. Do not rub after pulling back the needle and apply pressure with cotton swab.

Intradermal Injection

- It means injection of medicine within the skin
- Sites: Anterior aspect of forearm, skin over the deltiod
- Needle: 25 gauge
- Select an undamaged and uninfected area of skin. Stretch the skin between the thumb and forearm of one hand; with the other hand slowly insert the needle for about 2 mm just under and almost parallel to the surface of the skin. Considerable resistance is felt when injecting intradermally. A raised blenched bleb showing the surface of the hair follicles is a sign that the injection has been given correctly.

Administration of Oral Medication

- It means administering medicine into the oral passage
- Formulation available: Tablets, Capsules, Syrup, Drops etc.
- Devices: Various devices are available for measuring and administration of medicines i.e. measuring cups, small and large caliberated droppers, cylindrical spoons, oral syringes, measuring spoons etc.
- Conscious adults and older children can take tablets, capsules and liquid medicine using measuring devices themselves in sitting or is semirecumbent position. In younger children it can be given in sitting position

or in semi-recumbent position in mother's lap using measuring device as required. In patients with altered sensorium medicine should be given through feeding tube/ryles' tube.

Administration of Ophthalmic Medications

- Pre-requisites: Do not touch tip of the container or tip of cap. Warm the drop and ointment before using them by keeping at room temperature for few minutes
- Eye drops: Ask patient to lie supine on bed or sit on a chair with head tilted backwards and looking upwards. Then pull down the lower eyelid and instill drug into the space created between the eyelid and eyeball. Then ask the patient to slowly close the eye. Keep a gap of 5–7 minutes for second drop to be instilled
- Eye ointment: Squeeze 1 to 2 cm length ointment inside lower eyelid, then slowly close the eye and ask patient to roll closed eye in all directions. Keep a gap of 10–15 minutes for second ointment to be instilled.

Administration of Ear Medications

- Pre-requisites: Warm the ear drops before instilling
- Tilt the head just opposite to the ear to be used or make the patient lie in lateral position. In children < 3 years pull the ear downward and outward; > in 3 years and in adults pull the ear upwards and outwards then instill the required amount of drops. Keep the patient in same position for 5–10 minutes. A small amount of cotton can be placed in external canal if required.

Administration of Nasal Drops/Sprays

- Pre-requisites:
  - Nasal passage should be cleared of any secretions
  - If nasal passage is congested then decongestant can be used prior to drug
- Make the pateint lie supine and elevate chin or keep head upright, then instill the required amount of drug, keep him lie in the same position for few minutes.

Administration of Medications by Nebulizer

- Pre-requisites:
  - Check the electricity and nebulizer
  - Clean the mask or mouthpiece to be used
  - Mix/prepare medication as directed
  - Put medicine in the drug chamber, assemble mask or mouthpiece with chamber and connect it with tubing to port on compressor, then plug the machine

- Patient should be seated in upright position or in semi-recumbent position. Fit mask over nose and mouth or put mouthpiece into mouth and make sure that mist does not flow into eyes. Turn on compressor. Ask patient to take slow but deep breaths and continue nebulization until drug chamber is empty.

INDEX

C

D

K

L

M

N

O

P

Q

R

S

T

U

V

X

Z